ECG Interpretation

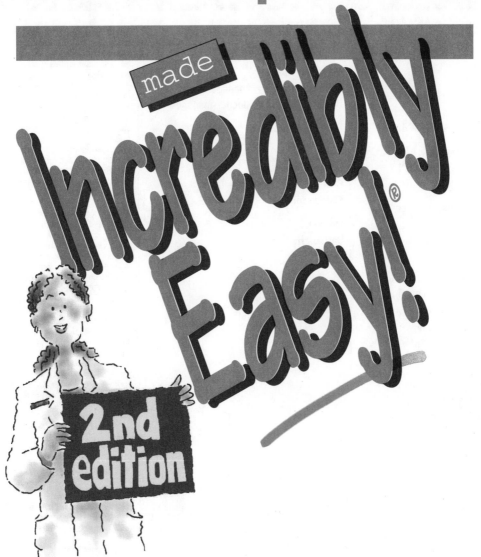

made Incredibly Easy!

2nd edition

Springhouse
Springhouse, Pennsylvania

Staff

Publisher
Judith A. Schilling McCann, RN, MSN

Executive Editor
Kate Jackson

Clinical Manager
Joan M. Robinson, RN, MSN, CCRN

Clinical Project Manager
Collette Bishop Hendler, RN, CCRN

Editors
Brenna Mayer (senior associate editor),
Cheryl Duksta, Ty Eggenberger,
Stacey Ann Follin, Kirk Robinson

Copy Editors
Jaime L. Stockslager (supervisor),
Virginia Baskerville, Kimberly Bilotta,
Priscilla DeWitt, Heather Ditch,
Amy Furman, Shana Harrington,
Malinda LaPrade, Dorothy P. Terry,
Pamela Wingrod, Helen Winton

Designers
Arlene Putterman (associate design
director), Mary Ludwicki (art director),
Lynn Foulk

Photographer
John Gallagher

Illustrators
Scott Thorn Barrows, Barbara Cousins,
John Cymerman, Mark Lefkowitz,
Judy Newhouse, Bot Roda, Mary Stangl,
Nina Wallace, Larry Ward

Electronic Production Services
Diane Paluba (manager), Joyce Rossi Biletz

Manufacturing
Patricia K. Dorshaw (manager),
Otto Mezei (book production manager)

Projects Coordinator
Liz Schaeffer

Editorial Assistants
Beverly Lane, Beth Janae Orr,
Elfriede Young

Indexer
Barbara Hodgson

The clinical treatments described and recommended in this publication are based on research and consultation with nursing, medical, and legal authorities. To the best of our knowledge, these procedures reflect currently accepted practice. Nevertheless, they can't be considered absolute and universal recommendations. For individual applications, all recommendations must be considered in light of the patient's clinical condition and, before administration of new or infrequently used drugs, in light of the latest package-insert information. The authors and publisher disclaim responsibility for any adverse effects resulting from the suggested procedures, from any undetected errors, or from the reader's misunderstanding of the text.

Printed in the United States of America.

IEECG2–D N O S A J
03 02 01   10 9 8 7 6 5 4 3 2 1

Library of Congress Cataloging-in-Publication Data

ECG interpretation made incredibly easy.— 2nd ed.
   p.; cm.
   Includes index.
   1. Electrocardiography.
   I. Springhouse Corporation
   [DNLM: 1. Electrocardiography—Nurses'
instruction. 2. Arrhythmia—Nurses' instruction.
WG 140 E172 2001]

RC683.5.E5 E256 2001
616.1'207547—dc21   2001020926
ISBN 1-58255-135-9 (alk. paper)

Contents

Contributors and consultants

Nancy J. Bekken, RN, MS, CCRN
Staff Educator, Adult Critical Care and
  Medical-Surgical Telemetry
Spectrum Health
Grand Rapids, Mich.

Christine Clayton, RN, MS, CNS, CNP
Nurse Practitioner
Cardiac Services
Sioux Valley Hospital
Sioux Falls, S. Dak.

Julene B. Kruithof, RN, MSN, CCRN
Staff Educator
Spectrum Health
Grand Rapids, Mich.

Amy M. Obermueller, RN, MSN, CCRN
Assistant Professor
Saint Luke's College
Kansas City, Mo.

L. M. Porterfield, RN, PhD
Director of Cardiovascular Research
Arrhythmia Consultants
Memphis

Ruthie Robinson, RN, MSN, CCRN, CEN
Instructor of Nursing
Lamar University
Beaumont, Tex.

Michelle Robinson-Jackson, MSN, CRNP, CS
Staff Nurse, Intensive Care Unit
Fox Chase Cancer Center
Philadelphia

Alexander John Siomko, RN,C, MSN, CRNP
Staff Nurse, Telemetry
Methodist Hospital Division, Thomas
  Jefferson University Hospital
Philadelphia

Mary A. Stahl, RN,CS, MSN, CCRN
Clinical Nurse Specialist
Saint Luke's Hospital
Kansas City, Mo.

Barbara A. Todd, MSN, CRNP
Director, Clinical Services Cardiac Surgery
Temple University Hospital
Philadelphia

*We extend special thanks to the
following people who contributed
to the previous edition:*

Deborah Becker, MSN, CRNP, CS, CCRN
Janice M. Beitz, RN, PhD, CS, CNOR, CETN
Lois M. Catts, RN, MSN, CCRN
Janet Davies-Choromanski, RN, MSN, CCRN, CS
Robin Donohoe Dennison, RN, MSN, CCRN, CS
Latrell P. Fowler, RN, PhD
Cynthia L. Hermey, RN, MN, CCRN
Peggy Jenkins, RN, MS, CCRN
Marsha Lowrie, RN, MS
Tamara Luedtke, RN, MSN, CCRN
Carol Lynn Maxwell-Thompson, RN, MSN, CCRN
Carrie A. McCoy, RN, MSN, CEN
Leanna R. Miller, RN, MSN, CCRN, CEN, CPNP
Patricia A. Mullins, RN, MS, CCRN
Christine Nicolai, RN, MS, CNS, CNP
Carla Roy, RN, BSN
Judith P. Vierke, RN, MS, CCRN

Foreword

It was my pleasure to contribute to the first edition of *ECG Interpretation Made Incredibly Easy*. At the time, I believed it would be impossible to top the first edition. Fortunately, I've been proven wrong.

ECG Interpretation Made Incredibly Easy, Second Edition, makes reading and understanding ECGs easier and more entertaining than you can imagine. Whether you're caring for a patient with an evolving myocardial infarction in the emergency room, a bypass patient in an intensive care unit, a knee-replacement patient on a medical-surgical floor, or a patient in your doctor's office, you need to quickly recognize and correctly react to common and uncommon arrhythmias. This book offers a step-by-step approach to accurate interpretation of arrhythmias.

ECG Interpretation Made Incredibly Easy, Second Edition, is divided into 12 chapters that cover the anatomy and physiology of the heart, how to obtain a high-quality rhythm strip, and how to correctly interpret all components of an ECG. You'll also learn how to help manage arrhythmias with the use of antiarrhythmic drugs, pacemakers, and implantable cardioverter-defibrillators. Scores of interesting rhythm strips and 12-lead ECGs give you a chance to really understand arrhythmias.

Each chapter includes a summary of key points at the beginning, plentiful cartoons that reinforce information to make learning fun and memorable, and a quick quiz at the end with plenty of practice strips to test what you've learned. Every chapter on arrhythmias covers the causes, signs and symptoms, and interventions for each arrhythmia.

Special logos throughout instantly draw your attention to the most important information. For example:

Don't skip this strip shows an ECG strip of every major arrhythmia with pointers on how to identify each one.

Mixed signals gives troubleshooting advice for equipment malfunction or unexpected ECG results.

This book is a wonderful reference designed for nurses, nurse practitioners, nursing students, and any other health care professionals who really want to master the field. The information is conveyed in a unique, lighthearted writing style that's both enjoyable and easy to understand.

This second edition features:
- completely updated information
- 25 additional rhythm strips and answer keys interspersed throughout the book to reinforce learning
- expanded coverage of antiarrhythmic drugs
- cheat sheets that highlight key points and provide the reader with a quick-study reference
- *Practice makes perfect* test at the end of the book that tests your overall knowledge with questions and answers in a true-to-life case-study format.

ECG Interpretation Made Incredibly Easy, Second Edition, provides a nonthreatening and effective learning experience. It's practical, clear, and fun to use. Every time you correctly interpret a simple or complex rhythm, you'll gain new confidence. You'll like this edition for its sheer sense of fun on a challenging subject!

Linda M. Porterfield, RN, PhD
Director of Cardiovascular Research
Arrhythmia Consultants, P.C.
Adjunct Assistant Professor
University of Tennessee
Memphis

Part I

ECG fundamentals

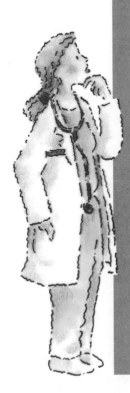

Cardiac anatomy and physiology

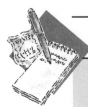

Just the facts

This chapter covers the structure of the heart and the coronary arteries, how the cardiac system works, and how arrhythmias affect a patient's well-being. In this chapter, you'll learn:

♦ about the location and structure of the heart

♦ about the layers of the heart wall

♦ how and through which structures blood flows to and through the heart

♦ what comprises the cardiac cycle and why understanding the cycle is important

♦ the properties of cardiac cells

♦ how impulse conduction works in the heart and how arrhythmias start.

A look at cardiac anatomy

Cardiac anatomy takes into account the location of the heart; the structure of the heart, heart wall, chambers, and valves; and the layout and structure of coronary circulation.

Outside the heart

The heart is a cone-shaped, muscular organ. It's located in the chest, behind the sternum in the mediastinal cavity (or mediastinum), between the lungs, and in front of the spine. (See *Where the heart lies*, page 11.) The heart lies tilted in this area, like an upside-down triangle. The top of the heart, or its base, lies just below the second rib; the bottom of the heart, or its apex, tilts for-

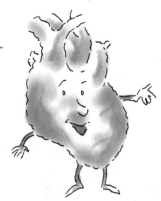

The mediastinum is home to the heart.

Layers of the heart wall

This cross section of the heart wall shows its various layers.

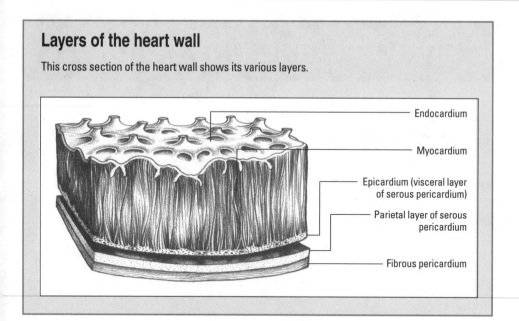

ward and down, toward the left side of the body, and rests on the diaphragm.

The heart varies in size depending on the person's body size, but the organ is roughly 5″ (12.5 cm) long and 3½″ (9 cm) wide, or about the size of the person's fist. The heart's weight, typically 9 to 12 oz (255 to 340 g), varies depending on the person's size, age, sex, and athletic conditioning. An athlete's heart usually weighs more than that of the average person, and an elderly person's heart weighs less.

Layer upon layer

The heart's wall is made up of three layers: the epicardium, myocardium, and endocardium. (See *Layers of the heart wall*.) The epicardium, the outer layer (and the visceral layer of the serous pericardium), is made up of squamous epithelial cells overlying connective tissue. The myocardium, the middle layer, makes up the largest portion of the heart's wall. This layer of muscle tissue contracts with each heartbeat. The endocardium, the heart's innermost layer, contains endothelial tissue with small blood vessels and bundles of smooth muscle.

A skeleton of connective tissue called the pericardium surrounds the heart and acts as a tough, protective sac. It consists of the fibrous pericardium and the serous pericardium. The fibrous pericardium, composed of tough, white, fibrous tis-

I rest on your diaphragm.

sue, fits loosely around the heart, protecting it. The serous pericardium, the thin, smooth, inner portion, has two layers:
• the parietal layer, which lines the inside of the fibrous pericardium
• the visceral layer, which adheres to the surface of the heart.

Between the layers

The pericardial space separates the visceral and parietal layers and contains 10 to 20 ml of thin, clear pericardial fluid that lubricates the two surfaces and cushions the heart. Excess pericardial fluid, a condition called pericardial effusion, can compromise the heart's ability to pump blood.

Inside the heart

The heart contains four chambers—two atria and two ventricles. (See *Inside a normal heart*, page 6.) The right and left atria serve as volume reservoirs for blood being sent into the ventricles. The right atrium receives deoxygenated blood returning from the body through the inferior and superior vena cavae and from the heart through the coronary sinus. The left atrium receives oxygenated blood from the lungs through the four pulmonary veins. The interatrial septum divides the chambers and helps them contract. Contraction of the atria forces blood into the ventricles below.

Pump up the volume

The right and left ventricles serve as the pumping chambers of the heart. The right ventricle receives blood from the right atrium and pumps it through the pulmonary arteries to the lungs, where it picks up oxygen and drops off carbon dioxide. The left ventricle receives oxygenated blood from the left atrium and pumps it through the aorta and then out to the rest of the body. The interventricular septum separates the ventricles and also helps them to pump.

The thickness of a chamber's walls depends on the amount of high-pressure work the chamber does. Because the atria collect blood for the ventricles and don't pump it far, their walls are considerably thinner than the walls of the ventricles. Likewise, the left ventricle has a much thicker wall than the right ventricle because the left ventricle pumps blood against the higher pressures in the body's arterial circulation, whereas the right ventricle pumps blood against the lower pressures in the lungs.

One-way valves

The heart contains four valves—two atrioventricular (AV) valves (tricuspid and mitral) and two semilunar valves (aortic and

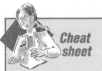

Cheat sheet

The heart's valves

• Tricuspid (AV valve between the right atrium and right ventricle)
• Mitral (AV valve between the left atrium and left ventricle)
• Aortic (semilunar valve between the left ventricle and the aorta)
• Pulmonic (semilunar valve between the right ventricle and the pulmonary artery)

Inside a normal heart

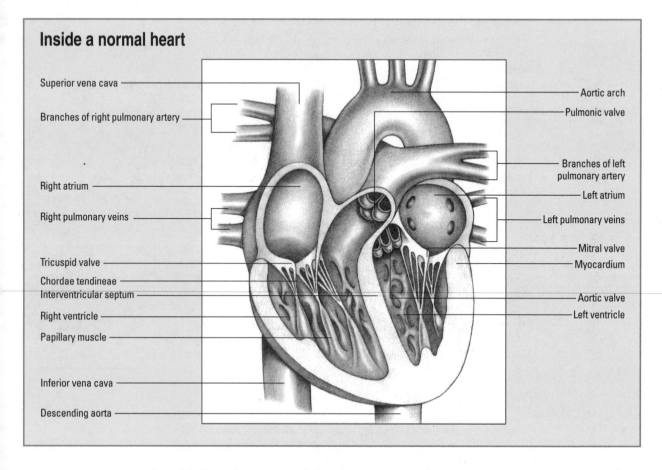

Superior vena cava

Branches of right pulmonary artery

Right atrium

Right pulmonary veins

Tricuspid valve

Chordae tendineae

Interventricular septum

Right ventricle

Papillary muscle

Inferior vena cava

Descending aorta

Aortic arch

Pulmonic valve

Branches of left pulmonary artery

Left atrium

Left pulmonary veins

Mitral valve

Myocardium

Aortic valve

Left ventricle

pulmonic). The valves open and close in response to changes in pressure within the chambers they connect and serve as one-way doors that keep blood flowing through the heart in a forward direction.

When the valves close, they prevent backflow, or regurgitation, of blood from one chamber to another. The closing of the valves creates the heart sounds heard through a stethoscope during a physical examination.

The two AV valves, located between the atria and ventricles, are called the tricuspid and mitral valves. The tricuspid valve is located between the right atrium and the right ventricle. The mitral valve is located between the left atrium and the left ventricle.

Cardiac cords

The mitral valve has two cusps, or leaflets, and the tricuspid valve has three. The cusps are anchored to the papillary muscles in the heart wall by fibers called chordae tendineae. These cords work together to prevent the cusps from bulging backward into the atria during ventricular contraction. Damage to them may allow blood to flow backward into a chamber, resulting in a heart murmur.

Cusps of the half-moons

The semilunar valves are the pulmonic valve and the aortic valve. These valves are called semilunar because the cusps resemble three half-moons. Because of the high pressures exerted on the valves, their structure is much simpler than that of the AV valves.

They open due to pressure within the ventricles and close due to the back pressure of blood in the pulmonary arteries and aorta, which pushes the cusps closed. The pulmonic valve, located where the pulmonary artery meets the right ventricle, permits blood to flow from the right ventricle to the pulmonary artery and prevents blood backflow into that ventricle. The aortic valve, located where the left ventricle meets the aorta, allows blood to flow from the left ventricle to the aorta and prevents blood backflow into the left ventricle.

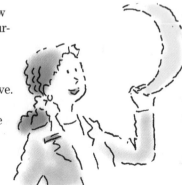

Blood flow through the heart

Understanding the flow of blood through the heart is critical for understanding the overall functions of the heart and how changes in electrical activity affect peripheral blood flow. Deoxygenated blood from the body returns to the heart through the inferior and superior vena cavae and empties into the right atrium. From there, blood flows through the tricuspid valve into the right ventricle.

Circuit city

The right ventricle pumps blood through the pulmonic valve into the pulmonary arteries and then into the lungs. From the lungs, blood flows through the pulmonary veins and empties into the left atrium, which completes a circuit called pulmonary circulation.

When pressure rises to a critical point in the left atrium, the mitral valve opens and blood flows into the left ventricle. The left ventricle then contracts and pumps blood through the aortic valve into the aorta, and then throughout the body. Blood returns to the right atrium through the veins, completing a circuit called systemic circulation.

Getting into circulation

Like the brain and all other organs, the heart needs an adequate supply of blood to survive. The coronary arteries, which lie on the surface of the heart, supply the heart muscle with blood and oxy-

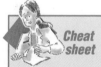

Cheat sheet

Blood flow

- Deoxygenated blood from the body returns to the right atrium and then flows to the right ventricle.
- The right ventricle pumps blood into the lungs where it's oxygenated. Then the blood returns to the left atrium and flows to the left ventricle.
- Oxygenated blood is pumped to the aorta and the body by the left ventricle.

gen. (See *The heart's vessels*, page 12.) Understanding coronary blood flow can help you provide better care for a patient with a myocardial infarction because you'll be able to predict which areas of the heart would be affected by a blockage in a particular coronary artery.

Open that ostium

The coronary ostium, an opening in the aorta that feeds blood to the coronary arteries, is located near the aortic valve. During systole, when the left ventricle is pumping blood through the aorta and the aortic valve is open, the coronary ostium is partially covered. During diastole, when the left ventricle is filling with blood, the aortic valve is closed and the coronary ostium is open, enabling blood to fill the coronary arteries.

With a shortened diastole, which occurs during periods of tachycardia, less blood flows through the ostium into the coronary arteries. Tachycardia also impedes coronary blood flow because contraction of the ventricles squeezes the arteries and lessens blood flow through them.

That's right, Coronary

The right coronary artery, as well as the left coronary artery (also known as the left main artery), originates as a single branch off the ascending aorta. The right coronary artery supplies blood to the right atrium, the right ventricle, and part of the inferior and posterior surfaces of the left ventricle. In about 50% of the population, the artery also supplies blood to the sinoatrial (SA) node. The bundle of His and the AV node also receive their blood supply from the right coronary artery.

What's left, Coronary?

The left coronary artery runs along the surface of the left atrium, where it splits into two major branches, the left anterior descending and the left circumflex arteries. The left anterior descending artery runs down the surface of the left ventricle toward the apex and supplies blood to the anterior wall of the left ventricle, the interventricular septum, the right bundle branch, and the left anterior fasciculus of the left bundle branch. The branches of the left anterior descending artery — the septal perforators and the diagonal arteries — help supply blood to the walls of both ventricles.

Circling circumflex

The circumflex artery supplies oxygenated blood to the lateral walls of the left ventricle, the left atrium and, in about half of the population, the SA node. In addition, the circumflex artery supplies blood to the left posterior fasciculus of the left bundle

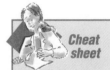

Cheat sheet

Arteries and veins

• *Right coronary artery* — supplies blood to the right atrium and ventricle and part of the left ventricle
• *Left anterior descending artery* — supplies blood to the anterior wall of the left ventricle, interventricular septum, right bundle branch, and left anterior fasciculus of the left bundle branch
• *Circumflex artery* — supplies blood to the lateral walls of the left ventricle, left atrium, and left posterior fasciculus of the bundle branch
• *Cardiac veins* — collect blood from the capillaries of the myocardium
• *Coronary sinus* — returns blood to the right atrium

branch. This artery circles around the left ventricle and provides blood to the ventricle's posterior portion.

Circulation, guaranteed

When two or more arteries supply the same region, they usually connect through anastomoses, junctions that provide alternative routes of blood flow. This network of smaller arteries, called collateral circulation, provides blood to capillaries that directly feed the heart muscle. Collateral circulation often becomes so strong that even if major coronary arteries become clogged with plaque, collateral circulation can continue to supply blood to the heart.

Veins in the heart

The heart has veins just like other parts of the body. Cardiac veins collect deoxygenated blood from the capillaries of the myocardium. The cardiac veins join together to form an enlarged vessel called the coronary sinus, which returns blood to the right atrium, where it continues through the circulation.

> **Quick facts about circulation**
>
> • It would take about 25 capillaries laid end-to-end to fill 1″ (2.5 cm).
> • The body contains about 10 billion capillaries.
> • On average, it takes a red blood cell less than 1 minute to travel from the heart to the capillaries and back again.

A look at cardiac physiology

This discussion of cardiac physiology includes descriptions of the cardiac cycle, how the cardiac muscle is innervated, how the depolarization-repolarization cycle operates, how impulses are conducted, and how abnormal impulses work. (See *Phases of the cardiac cycle*, page 10.)

Cardiac cycle dynamics

During one heartbeat, ventricular diastole (relaxation) and ventricular systole (contraction) occur.

During diastole, the ventricles relax, the atria contract, and blood is forced through the open tricuspid and mitral valves. The aortic and pulmonic valves are closed.

During systole, the atria relax and fill with blood. The mitral and tricuspid valves are closed. Ventricular pressure rises, which forces open the aortic and pulmonic valves. Then the ventricles contract, and blood flows through the circulatory system.

Atrial kick

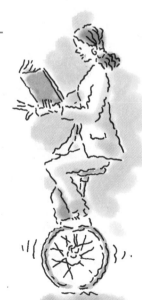

The atrial contraction, or atrial kick, contributes about 30% of the cardiac output—the amount of blood pumped by the ventricles in 1 minute. (See *Quick facts about circulation.*) Certain arrhythmias, such as atrial fibrillation, can cause a loss of atrial kick and

Phases of the cardiac cycle

The cardiac cycle consists of the following phases.

1. *Isovolumetric ventricular contraction.* In response to ventricular depolarization, tension in the ventricles increases. The rise in pressure within the ventricles leads to closure of the mitral and tricuspid valves. The pulmonic and aortic valves stay closed during the entire phase.

2. *Ventricular ejection.* When ventricular pressure exceeds aortic and pulmonary arterial pressure, the aortic and pulmonic valves open and the ventricles eject blood.

3. *Isovolumetric relaxation.* When ventricular pressure falls below pressure in the aorta and pulmonary artery, the aortic and pulmonic valves close. All valves are closed during this phase. Atrial diastole occurs as blood fills the atria.

4. *Ventricular filling.* Atrial pressure exceeds ventricular pressure, which causes the mitral and tricuspid valves to open. Blood then flows passively into the ventricles. About 70% of ventricular filling takes place during this phase.

5. *Atrial systole.* Known as the atrial kick, atrial systole (coinciding with late ventricular diastole) supplies the ventricles with the remaining 30% of the blood for each heartbeat.

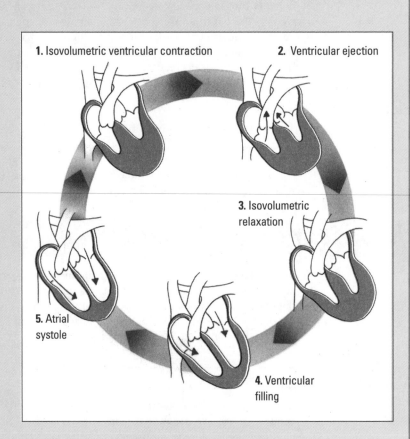

1. Isovolumetric ventricular contraction

2. Ventricular ejection

3. Isovolumetric relaxation

4. Ventricular filling

5. Atrial systole

a subsequent drop in cardiac output. Tachycardia also affects cardiac output by shortening diastole and allowing less time for the ventricles to fill. Less filling time means less blood will be ejected during ventricular systole and less will be sent through the circulation.

(Text continues on page 15.)

Where the heart lies

This illustration shows exactly where the heart is located. The heart lies within the mediastinum, a cavity that contains the tissues and organs separating the two pleural sacs. In most people, two-thirds of the heart extends to the left of the body's midline.

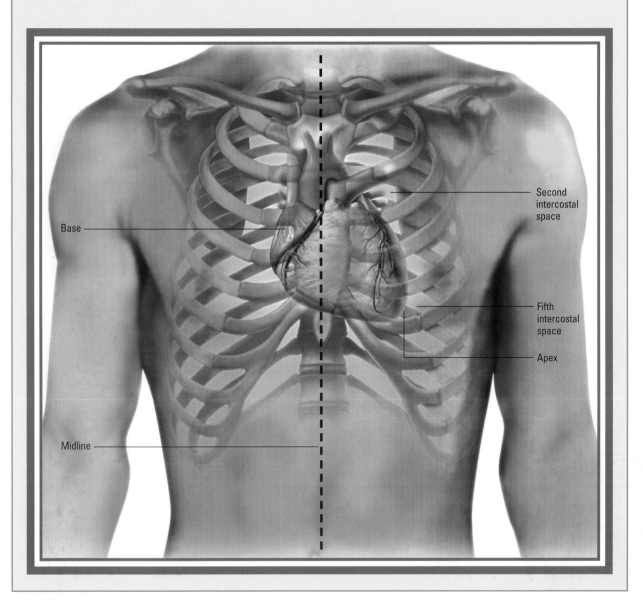

The heart's vessels

The two views of the heart shown below detail the great vessels and some of the major coronary vessels.

ANTERIOR VIEW

POSTERIOR VIEW

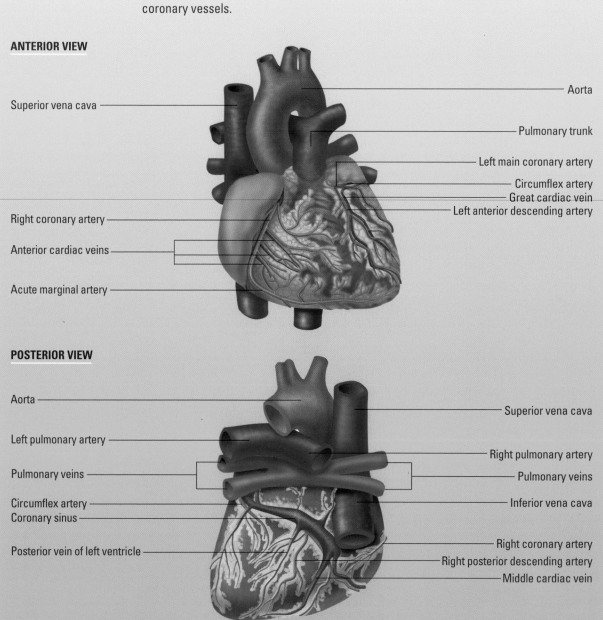

Anterior view labels:
- Superior vena cava
- Aorta
- Pulmonary trunk
- Left main coronary artery
- Circumflex artery
- Great cardiac vein
- Left anterior descending artery
- Right coronary artery
- Anterior cardiac veins
- Acute marginal artery

Posterior view labels:
- Aorta
- Superior vena cava
- Left pulmonary artery
- Right pulmonary artery
- Pulmonary veins
- Pulmonary veins
- Circumflex artery
- Inferior vena cava
- Coronary sinus
- Posterior vein of left ventricle
- Right coronary artery
- Right posterior descending artery
- Middle cardiac vein

Conducting impulses

The conduction system of the heart, shown below, begins with the heart's pacemaker, the sinoatrial (SA) node. When an impulse leaves the SA node, it travels through the atria along Bachmann's bundle and the internodal pathways on its way to the atrioventricular (AV) node and the ventricles.

After the impulse passes through the AV node, it travels to the ventricles, first down the bundle of His, then along the bundle branches and, finally, down the Purkinje fibers.

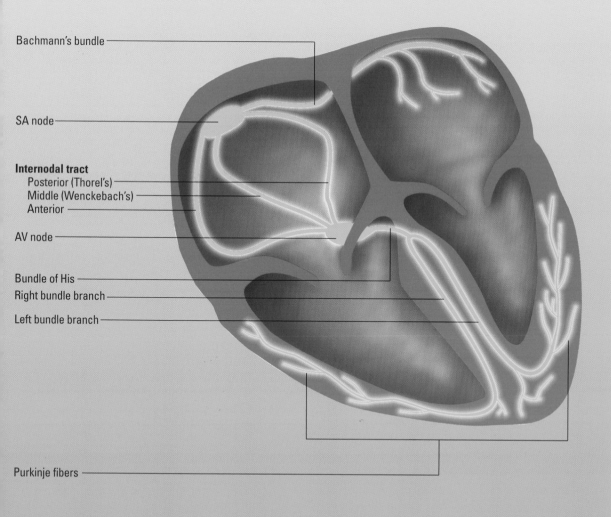

Bachmann's bundle

SA node

Internodal tract
   Posterior (Thorel's)
   Middle (Wenckebach's)
   Anterior

AV node

Bundle of His

Right bundle branch

Left bundle branch

Purkinje fibers

How reentry develops

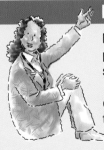

Normally, conduction occurs along a single pathway, so reentry can't occur. In some people, however, conduction occurs along two pathways — one fast and one slow. The speed and frequency of impulse conduction varies along those paths.

Think of the two pathways as racetracks. One track has a perfect surface for speed. The other meanders through an obstacle course. An impulse starting off stays together until the tracks diverge.

Unidirectional conduction

At that point, the impulse — like a group of runners — splits up, as shown on the right. Half of them take the fast track, and half struggle through obstacles on the slow track. The fast-track runners reach the finish line well ahead of the slow-track runners, which causes the slow-track runners to stop running and disperse.

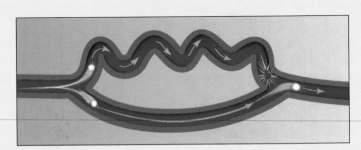

Premature impulse

If an ectopic impulse reaches the tracks earlier than usual, the fast track isn't ready; it's still refractory from the previous conduction. In such cases, as shown on the left, the impulse takes the slow track, which can accept runners more quickly.

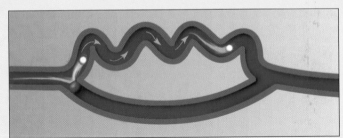

Reentry

When the runners reach the bottom of the slow track, as shown on the right, one runner splits off and heads to the finish line. The others are so excited that they head back up the fast track in a kind of victory lap. The impulse then continues around the circuit — down the slow track and up the fast track — repeatedly, sending one runner each time to the finish line and one back up to the starting point. That continuous looping of an impulse through the two pathways, known as reentry, can result in tachyarrhythmias.

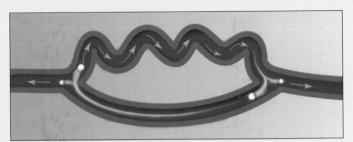

Your cycle's output

The cardiac cycle produces cardiac output, which is the amount of blood the heart pumps in 1 minute. It's measured by multiplying heart rate times stroke volume. (See *Preload and afterload,* page 16.) The term stroke volume refers to the amount of blood ejected with each ventricular contraction.

Normal cardiac output is 4 to 8 L per minute, depending on body size. The heart pumps only as much blood as the body requires. Three factors affect stroke volume—preload, afterload, and myocardial contractility. A balance of these three factors produces optimal cardiac output.

Preload

Preload is the stretching of muscle fibers in the ventricles and is determined by the pressure and amount of blood remaining in the left ventricle at the end of diastole.

Afterload

Afterload is the amount of pressure the left ventricle must work against to pump blood into the circulation. The greater this resistance, the more the heart works to pump out blood.

Contractility

Contractility is the ability of muscle cells to contract after depolarization. This ability depends on how much the muscle fibers are stretched at the end of diastole.

Overstretching or understretching these fibers alters contractility and the amount of blood pumped out of the ventricles. Picture trying to shoot a rubber band across the room. If you don't stretch it enough, it won't go far. If you stretch it too much, it will snap. However, if you stretch it just the right amount, it will go as far as you want it to.

Nerve supply to the heart

The heart is supplied by the two branches of the autonomic nervous system—the sympathetic (or adrenergic) and the parasympathetic (or cholinergic).

The sympathetic nervous system is basically the heart's accelerator. Two sets of chemicals—norepinephrine and epinephrine—are highly influenced by this system. These chemicals increase heart rate, automaticity, atrioventricular conduction, and contractility.

Preload and afterload

Preload refers to a passive stretching exerted by blood on the ventricular muscle at the end of diastole. According to Starling's law, the more the cardiac muscles are stretched in diastole, the more forcefully they contract in systole.

Afterload refers to the pressure that the ventricles need to generate to overcome higher pressure in the aorta. Normally, pressure in the left ventricle at the end of diastole is 5 to 10 mm Hg. In the aorta, it's 70 to 80 mm Hg. That difference means that the left ventricle needs to pump with enough force to pop open the aortic valve.

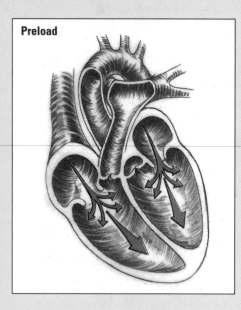

Preload

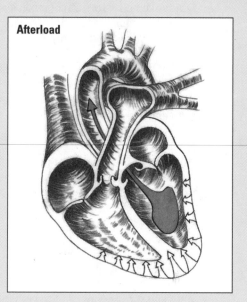

Afterload

Braking the heart

The parasympathetic nervous system, on the other hand, serves as the heart's brakes. One of this system's nerves, the vagus nerve, carries impulses that slow heart rate and the conduction of impulses through the AV node and ventricles. The vagus nerve is stimulated by baroreceptors, specialized nerve cells in the aorta and the internal carotid arteries. Things that stimulate the baroreceptors also stimulate the vagus nerve to apply its cardiac brakes.

For instance, a stretching of the baroreceptors—which can occur during periods of hypertension or when applying pressure to the carotid artery—stimulates the receptors. In a maneuver called carotid sinus massage, baroreceptors in the carotid arteries are purposely activated in an effort to slow a rapid heart rate.

Transmission of electrical impulses

The heart can't pump unless an electrical stimulus occurs first. Generation and transmission of electrical impulses depend on the automaticity, excitability, conductivity, and contractility of cardiac cells.

Terms revisited

The term automaticity refers to a cell's ability to spontaneously initiate an impulse. Pacemaker cells possess this ability. Excitability results from ion shifts across the cell membrane and indicates how well a cell responds to an electrical stimulus.

Conductivity is the ability of a cell to transmit an electrical impulse to another cardiac cell. Contractility refers to how well the cell contracts after receiving a stimulus.

"De"-cycle and "re"-cycle

As impulses are transmitted, cardiac cells undergo cycles of depolarization and repolarization. (See *Depolarization-repolarization cycle*, page 18.) Cardiac cells at rest are considered polarized, meaning that no electrical activity takes place. Cell membranes separate different concentrations of ions, such as sodium and potassium, and create a more negative charge inside the cell. This is called the resting potential. After a stimulus occurs, ions cross the cell membrane and cause an action potential, or cell depolarization.

When a cell is fully depolarized, it attempts to return to its resting state in a process called repolarization. Electrical charges in the cell reverse and return to normal.

A cycle of depolarization-repolarization consists of five phases—0 through 4. The action potential is represented by a curve that shows voltage changes during the five phases. (See *Action potential curve*, page 19.)

Many phases of the curve

During phase 0, the cell receives an impulse from a neighboring cell and is depolarized. Phase 1 is marked by early, rapid repolarization. Phase 2, the plateau phase, is a period of slow repolarization.

During phases 1 and 2 and at the beginning of phase 3, the cardiac cell is said to be in its absolute refractory period. During that period, no stimulus, no matter how strong, can excite the cell.

Phase 3, the rapid repolarization phase, occurs as the cell returns to its original state. During the last half of this phase, when the cell is in its relative refractory period, a very strong stimulus can depolarize it.

Depolarization-repolarization cycle

Use this illustration to review the five phases of the depolarization-repolarization cycle.

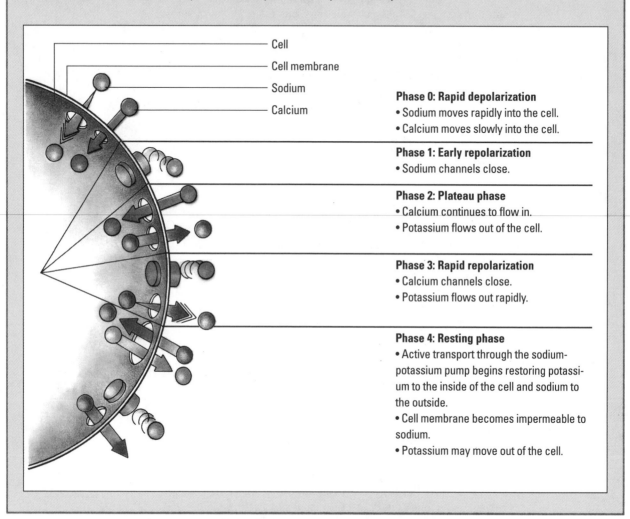

Cell

Cell membrane

Sodium

Calcium

Phase 0: Rapid depolarization
- Sodium moves rapidly into the cell.
- Calcium moves slowly into the cell.

Phase 1: Early repolarization
- Sodium channels close.

Phase 2: Plateau phase
- Calcium continues to flow in.
- Potassium flows out of the cell.

Phase 3: Rapid repolarization
- Calcium channels close.
- Potassium flows out rapidly.

Phase 4: Resting phase
- Active transport through the sodium-potassium pump begins restoring potassium to the inside of the cell and sodium to the outside.
- Cell membrane becomes impermeable to sodium.
- Potassium may move out of the cell.

Phase 4 is the resting phase of the action potential. By the end of phase 4, the cell is ready for another stimulus.

All that electrical activity is represented on an electrocardiogram (ECG). Keep in mind that the ECG represents electrical activity only, not actual pumping of the heart.

Action potential curve

An action potential curve shows the electrical changes in a myocardial cell during the depolarization-repolarization cycle. This graph shows the changes in a nonpacemaker cell.

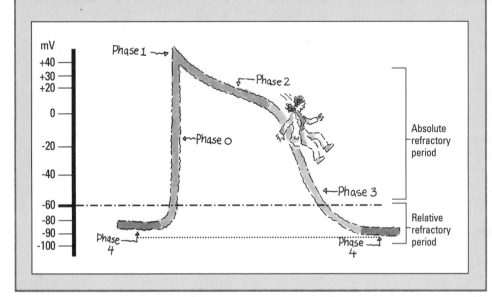

Pathway through the heart

After depolarization and repolarization occur, the resulting electrical impulse travels through the heart along a pathway called the conduction system. (See *Conducting impulses*, page 13.)

Impulses travel out from the SA node and through the internodal tracts and Bachmann's bundle to the AV node. From there, they travel through the bundle of His, the bundle branches, and finally to the Purkinje fibers.

Numero uno node

The SA node—located in the upper right corner of the right atrium where the superior vena cava joins the atrial tissue mass—is the heart's main pacemaker, generating impulses 60 to 100 times per minute. When initiated, the impulses follow a specific path through the heart. They usually can't flow in a backward direction because the cells can't respond to a stimulus immediately after depolarization.

Those impulses really get around!

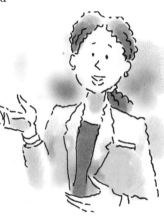

Bachmann's bundle of nerves

Impulses from the SA node next travel through Bachmann's bundle, tracts of tissue extending from the SA node to the left atrium. Impulses are thought to be transmitted throughout the right atrium through the anterior, middle, and posterior internodal tracts. Whether those tracts actually exist, however, is unclear. Impulse transmission through the right and left atria occurs so rapidly that the atria contract almost simultaneously.

AV: The slow node

The AV node, located in the inferior right atrium near the ostium of the coronary sinus, is responsible for delaying the impulses that reach it. Although the nodal tissue itself has no pacemaker cells, the tissue surrounding it (called junctional tissue) contains pacemaker cells that can fire at a rate of 40 to 60 times per minute.

The AV node's main function is to delay impulses by 0.04 second to keep the ventricles from contracting too quickly. This delay allows the ventricles to complete their filling phase as the atria contract. It also allows the cardiac muscle to stretch to its fullest for peak cardiac output.

Branch splitting

The bundle of His, a tract of tissue extending into the ventricles next to the interventricular septum, resumes the rapid conduction of the impulse through the ventricles. The bundle eventually divides into the right and left bundle branches.

The right bundle branch extends down the right side of the interventricular septum and through the right ventricle. The left bundle branch extends down the left side of the interventricular septum and through the left ventricle.

The left bundle branch then splits into two branches, or fasciculi: the left anterior fasciculus, which extends through the anterior portion of the left ventricle, and the left posterior fasciculus, which runs through the lateral and posterior portions of the left ventricle. Impulses travel much faster down the left bundle branch (which feeds the larger, thicker-walled left ventricle) than the right bundle branch (which feeds the smaller, thinner-walled right ventricle).

The difference in the conduction speed allows both ventricles to contract simultaneously. The entire network of specialized nervous tissue that extends through the ventricles is known as the His-Purkinje system.

Those perky Purkinje fibers

Purkinje fibers extend from the bundle branches into the endocardium, deep into the myocardial tissue. These fibers conduct

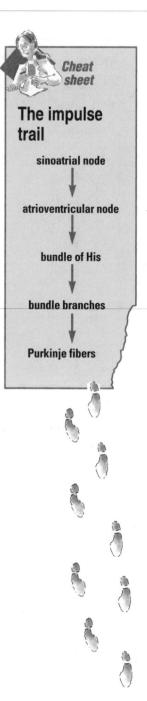

Cheat sheet

The impulse trail

sinoatrial node

↓

atrioventricular node

↓

bundle of His

↓

bundle branches

↓

Purkinje fibers

impulses rapidly through the muscle to assist in its depolarization and contraction.

Purkinje fibers can also serve as a pacemaker and are able to discharge impulses at a rate of 20 to 40 times per minute, sometimes even more slowly. (See *Pacemakers of the heart.*) Purkinje fibers usually aren't activated as a pacemaker unless conduction through the bundle of His becomes blocked or a higher pacemaker (SA or AV node) doesn't generate an impulse.

Abnormal impulses

Now that you understand how the heart generates a normal impulse, let's look at some causes of abnormal impulse conduction, including automaticity, backward conduction of impulses, reentry abnormalities, and ectopy.

When the heart goes on "manual"

Automaticity is a special characteristic of pacemaker cells to generate impulses automatically, without being stimulated to do so. If a cell's automaticity is increased or decreased, an arrhythmia can occur. Tachycardia, for instance, is commonly caused by an in-

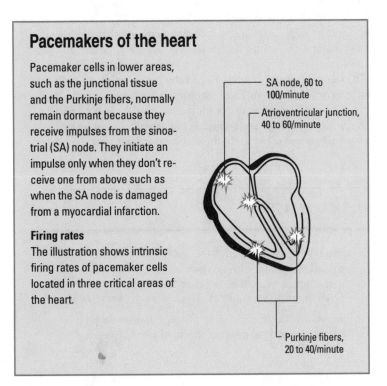

Pacemakers of the heart

Pacemaker cells in lower areas, such as the junctional tissue and the Purkinje fibers, normally remain dormant because they receive impulses from the sinoatrial (SA) node. They initiate an impulse only when they don't receive one from above such as when the SA node is damaged from a myocardial infarction.

Firing rates
The illustration shows intrinsic firing rates of pacemaker cells located in three critical areas of the heart.

SA node, 60 to 100/minute

Atrioventricular junction, 40 to 60/minute

Purkinje fibers, 20 to 40/minute

crease in the automaticity of pacemaker cells below the SA node. Likewise, a decrease in automaticity of cells in the SA node can cause the development of bradycardia or an escape rhythm (a compensatory beat generated by a lower pacemaker site).

Out of synch

Impulses that begin below the AV node can be transmitted backward toward the atria. This backward, or retrograde, conduction usually takes longer than normal conduction and can cause the atria and ventricles to beat out of synch.

Coming back for more

Sometimes impulses cause depolarization twice in a row at a faster-than-normal rate. Such events are referred to as reentry events. In reentry, impulses are delayed long enough that cells have time to repolarize. (See *How reentry develops*, page 14.) In these cases, the active impulse reenters the same area and produces another impulse.

Repeating itself

An injured pacemaker (or nonpacemaker) cell may partially depolarize, rather than fully depolarizing. Partial depolarization can lead to spontaneous or secondary depolarization, repetitive ectopic firings called triggered activity.

The resultant depolarization is called afterdepolarization. Early afterdepolarization occurs before the cell is fully repolarized and can be caused by hypokalemia, slow pacing rates, or drug toxicity. If it occurs after the cell has been fully repolarized, it's called delayed afterdepolarization. These problems can be caused by digoxin toxicity, hypercalcemia, or increased catecholamine release. Atrial or ventricular tachycardias may result. You'll learn more about these and other arrhythmias in later chapters.

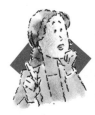

Quick quiz

1. The term automaticity refers to the ability of a cell to:
    A.   initiate an impulse on its own.
    B.   send impulses in all directions.
    C.   block impulses formed in areas other than the SA node.

Answer: A. Automaticity, the ability of a cell to initiate an impulse on its own, is a unique characteristic of cardiac cells.

2. Parasympathetic stimulation of the heart results in:
- A. increased heart rate and slower AV conduction.
- B. increased heart rate and faster AV conduction.
- C. decreased heart rate and slower AV conduction.

Answer: C. Parasympathetic stimulation of the vagus nerve causes a decrease in heart rate and slowed AV conduction.

3. The normal pacemaker of the heart is the:
- A. SA node.
- B. AV node.
- C. bundle of His.

Answer: A. The SA node is the main pacemaker of the heart, firing at an intrinsic rate of 60 to 100 times per minute.

4. The impulse delay produced by the AV node allows the atria to:
- A. repolarize simultaneously.
- B. contract before the ventricles.
- C. send impulses to the bundle of His.

Answer: B. The 0.04-second delay allows the atria to contract and the ventricles to completely fill, which optimizes cardiac output.

5. The coronary arteries fill with blood during:
- A. atrial systole.
- B. atrial diastole.
- C. ventricular diastole.

Answer: C. The coronary arteries fill with blood when the ventricles are in diastole and filling with blood. The aortic valve is closed at that time, so it no longer blocks blood flow through the coronary ostium into the coronary arteries.

6. When stimulated, baroreceptors cause the heart rate to:
- A. increase.
- B. decrease.
- C. stay the same.

Answer: B. Baroreceptors, when stimulated, cause the heart rate to decrease.

7. The two valves called the semilunar valves are the:
- A. pulmonic and mitral valves.
- B. pulmonic and aortic valves.
- C. aortic and mitral valves.

Answer: B. The semilunar valves are the pulmonic and aortic valves.

8.   Passive stretching exerted by blood on the ventricular muscle at the end of diastole is referred to as:

    A.   preload.

    B.   afterload.

    C.   the atrial kick.

Answer: A. The passive stretching exerted by blood on the ventricular muscle at the end of diastole is called preload. It increases with an increase in venous return to the heart.

9.   Your patient who was admitted with an acute myocardial infarction develops a heart rate of 36 beats/minute. Based on this finding, which area of the patient's heart is most likely functioning as the pacemaker?

    A.   SA node

    B.   AV node

    C.   Purkinje fibers

Answer: C. The SA node is the heart's normal pacemaker. It fires at a rate of 60 to 100 beats/minute. When the SA node becomes damaged, the AV node takes over firing at 40 to 60 beats/minute. If this site also becomes damaged, the Purkinje fibers take over firing at a rate of 20 to 40 beats/minute.

Scoring

☆☆☆ If you answered all nine questions correctly, hooray! You're a happenin', heart-smart hipster!

☆☆ If you answered six to eight questions correctly, way to go! You're clearly heart smart!

☆ If you answered fewer than six questions correctly, take heart. Just review this chapter and you'll be up to speed.

2

Obtaining a rhythm strip

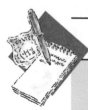

Just the facts

An ECG can be used to help diagnose cardiac and noncardiac illnesses and to monitor the effects of medications or electrolyte imbalances. In this chapter, you'll learn:

♦ how important the ECG is for providing effective patient care

♦ how leads and planes function

♦ what types of ECG monitoring systems are available

♦ how to apply electrodes, select leads, and obtain rhythm strips

♦ how to solve cardiac-monitoring problems.

A look at ECG recordings

The heart's electrical activity produces currents that radiate through the surrounding tissue to the skin. When electrodes are attached to the skin, they sense those electrical currents and transmit them to an electrocardiograph (ECG) monitor. The currents are then transformed into waveforms that represent the heart's depolarization-repolarization cycle.

You might remember that myocardial depolarization occurs when a wave of stimulation passes through the heart and causes the heart muscle to contract. Repolarization is the relaxation phase.

An ECG shows the precise sequence of electrical events occurring in the cardiac cells throughout that process. It allows the nurse to monitor phases of myocardial contraction and to identify rhythm and conduction disturbances. A series of ECGs can be used as a baseline comparison to assess cardiac function.

Leads and planes

To understand electrocardiography, you need to understand leads and planes. Electrodes placed on the skin measure the direction of electrical current discharged by the heart. That current is then transformed into waveforms.

An ECG records information about those waveforms from different views or perspectives. Those perspectives are called leads and planes.

> Leads and planes offer different views of the heart's electrical activity

Take the lead

A lead provides a view of the heart's electrical activity between one positive pole and one negative pole. Between the two poles lies an imaginary line representing the lead's axis, a term that refers to the direction of the current moving through the heart.

The direction of the current affects the direction in which the waveform points on an ECG. (See *Current direction and wave deflection.*) When no electrical activity occurs or the activity is too weak to measure, the waveform looks like a straight line, called an isoelectric waveform.

Current direction and wave deflection

The illustration shows possible directions of electrical current, or depolarization, on a lead. The direction of the electrical current determines the upward or downward deflection of an electrocardiogram waveform.

As current travels toward the negative pole, the waveform deflects mostly downward.

When current flows perpendicular to the lead, the waveform may be small or go in both directions (biphasic).

As current travels toward the positive pole, the waveform deflects mostly upward.

Plane and simple

The term "plane" refers to a cross-sectional perspective of the heart's electrical activity. The frontal plane, a vertical cut through the middle of the heart, provides an anterior-to-posterior view of electrical activity. The horizontal plane, a transverse cut through the middle of heart, provides either a superior or an inferior view.

Types of ECGs

The two types of ECG recordings are the 12-lead ECG and the single-lead ECG, commonly known as a rhythm strip. Both types give valuable information about heart function.

A dozen views

A 12-lead ECG records information from 12 different views of the heart and provides a complete picture of electrical activity. These 12 views are obtained by placing electrodes on the patient's limbs and chest. The limb leads and the chest, or precordial, leads reflect information from the different planes of the heart.

Different leads provide different information. The six limb leads—I, II, III, augmented vector right (aV_R), augmented vector left (aV_L), and augmented vector foot (aV_F)—provide information about the heart's frontal plane. Leads I, II, and III require a negative and positive electrode for monitoring, which makes those leads bipolar. The augmented leads record information from one lead and are called unipolar.

The six precordial or V leads—V_1, V_2, V_3, V_4, V_5, and V_6—provide information about the heart's horizontal plane. Like the augmented leads, the precordial leads are also unipolar, requiring only a single electrode. The opposing pole of those leads is the center of the heart as calculated by the ECG.

Just one view

Single-lead monitoring provides continuous information about the heart's electrical activity and is used to monitor cardiac status. Chest electrodes pick up the heart's electrical activity for display on the monitor. The monitor also displays heart rate and other measurements and prints out strips of cardiac rhythms.

Commonly monitored leads include the bipolar leads I, II, and III and two unipolar leads called MCL_1 and MCL_6. The initials MCL stand for modified chest lead. These leads are similar to the unipolar leads V_1 and V_6 of the 12-lead ECG. MCL_1 and MCL_6, however, are bipolar leads.

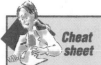

Cheat sheet

The 12-lead ECG

6 limb leads
• Provide information about the heart's frontal plane
• Bipolar (leads I, II, and III) because they require a negative and positive electrode for monitoring
• Unipolar (leads aV_R, aV_L, and aV_F) because they record information from one lead

6 precordial leads (leads V_1 through V_6)
• Provide information about the heart's horizontal plane
• Unipolar because they require only one electrode

Monitoring ECGs

The type of ECG monitoring system you'll use — hardwire monitoring or telemetry — depends on the patient's condition and the area in which you work. Let's look at each system.

Hardwire basics

With hardwire monitoring, the electrodes are connected directly to the cardiac monitor. Most hardwire monitors are mounted permanently on a shelf or wall near the patient's bed. Some monitors are mounted on an I.V. pole for portability, and some may include a defibrillator.

The monitor provides a continuous cardiac rhythm display and transmits the ECG tracing to a console at the nurses' station. Both the monitor and the console have alarms and can print rhythm strips to show ectopic beats, for instance, or other arrhythmias. Hardwire monitors can also track pulse oximetry, blood pressure, hemodynamic measurements, and other parameters through various attachments to the patient.

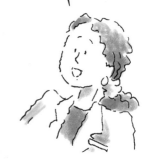

There are pros and cons with both monitoring systems.

Some drawbacks

Hardwire monitoring is generally used in critical care units and emergency departments because it permits continuous observation of one or more patients from more than one area in the unit. However, this type of monitoring does have drawbacks, among them:
• limited patient mobility because the patient is tethered to a monitor by electrodes
• patient discomfort because of the electrodes and cables attached to the chest
• possibility of lead disconnection and loss of cardiac monitoring when the patient moves
• accidental shock to the patient (rare).

Portable points

With telemetry monitoring, the patient carries a small, battery-powered transmitter that sends electrical signals to another location, where the signals are displayed on a monitor screen. This type of ECG monitoring frees the patient from cumbersome wires and cables and protects him from the electrical leakage and accidental shock occasionally associated with hardwire monitoring.

Telemetry monitoring still requires skin electrodes to be placed on the patient's chest. Each electrode is connected by a thin wire to a small transmitter box carried in a pocket or pouch.

Telemetry monitoring is especially useful for detecting arrhythmias that occur at rest or during sleep, exercise, or stressful situations. Most systems, however, can monitor heart rate and rhythm only.

All about leads

Electrode placement is different for each lead, and different leads provide different views of the heart. A lead may be chosen to highlight a particular part of the ECG complex or the electrical events of a specific cardiac cycle.

Although leads II, MCL_1, and MCL_6 are among the most commonly used leads for monitoring, you should adjust the leads according to the patient's condition. If your monitoring system has the capability, you may also monitor the patient in more than one lead. (See *Dual lead monitoring.*)

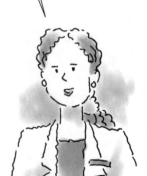

Adjust the leads according to the patient's condition.

Dual lead monitoring

Monitoring in two leads provides a more complete picture than monitoring in one. With simultaneous dual monitoring, you'll generally review the first lead—usually designated as the primary lead—for arrhythmias.

A two-lead view helps detect ectopic beats or aberrant rhythms. Leads II and V_1 are the leads most commonly monitored simultaneously.

Lead II

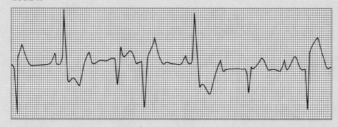

Lead V_1

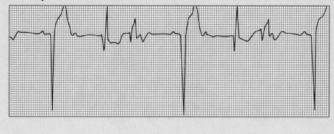

Going to ground

All bipolar leads have a third electrode, known as the ground, which is placed on the chest to prevent electrical interference from appearing on the ECG recording.

Heeeere's lead I

Lead I provides a view of the heart that shows current moving from right to left. Because current flows from negative to positive, the positive electrode for this lead is placed on the left arm or on the left side of the chest; the negative electrode is placed on the right arm. Lead I produces a positive deflection on ECG tracings and is helpful in monitoring atrial rhythms and hemiblocks.

Introducing lead II

Lead II produces a positive deflection. Place the positive electrode on the patient's left leg and the negative electrode on the right arm. For continuous monitoring, place the electrodes on the torso

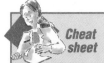

Cheat sheet

Leads I, II, and III

• *Leads I, II, and III* — typically produce positive deflection on electrocardiogram tracings
• *Lead I* — helpful in monitoring atrial rhythms and hemiblocks
• *Lead II* — commonly used for routine monitoring and detecting sinus node and atrial arrhythmias
• *Lead III* — useful for detecting changes associated with inferior wall myocardial infarction

Einthoven's triangle

When setting up standard limb leads, you'll place electrodes in positions commonly referred to as Einthoven's triangle, shown here. The electrodes for leads I, II, and III are about equidistant from the heart and form an equilateral triangle.

Axes

The axis of lead I extends from shoulder to shoulder, with the right-arm electrode being the negative electrode and the left-arm electrode positive.

The axis of lead II runs from the negative right-arm electrode to the positive left-leg electrode. The axis of lead III extends from the negative left-arm electrode to the left-leg electrode.

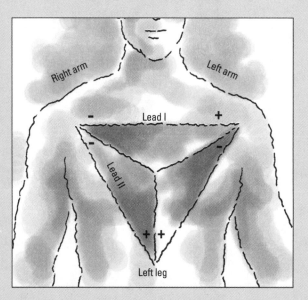

for convenience, with the positive electrode below the lowest palpable rib at the left midclavicular line and the negative electrode below the right clavicle. The current travels down and to the left in this lead. Lead II tends to produce a positive, high-voltage deflection, resulting in tall P, R, and T waves. This lead is commonly used for routine monitoring and is useful for detecting sinus node and atrial arrhythmias.

Next up, lead III

Lead III produces a positive deflection. The positive electrode is placed on the left leg; the negative electrode, on the left arm. Along with lead II, this lead is useful for detecting changes associated with an inferior wall myocardial infarction.

The axes of the three bipolar limb leads—I, II, and III—form a triangle around the heart and provide a frontal plane view of the heart. (See *Einthoven's triangle*.)

The "a" leads

Leads aV$_R$, aV$_L$, and aV$_F$ are called augmented leads because the small waveforms that normally would appear from these unipolar leads are enhanced by the ECG. (See *Augmented leads*.) The "a" stands for "augmented," and "R, L, and F" stand for the positive electrode position of the lead.

Augmented leads

Leads aV$_R$, aV$_L$, and aV$_F$ are called augmented leads. They measure electrical activity between one limb and a single electrode. Lead aV$_R$ provides no specific view of the heart. Lead aV$_L$ shows electrical activity coming from the heart's lateral wall. Lead aV$_F$ shows electrical activity coming from the heart's inferior wall.

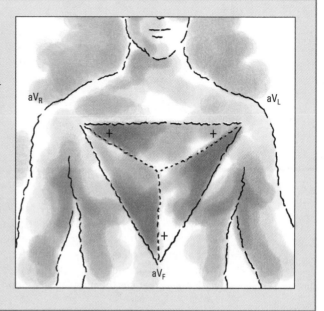

Precordial views

These illustrations show the different views of the heart obtained from each precordial (chest) lead.

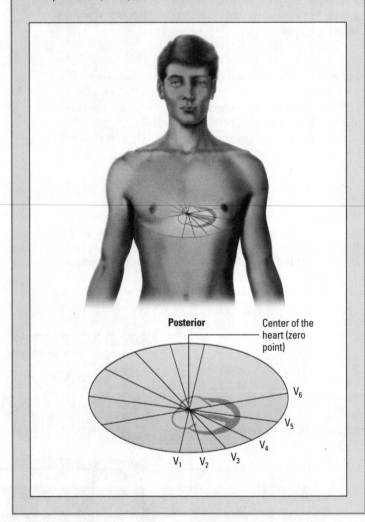

Posterior

Center of the heart (zero point)

V_6

V_5

V_4

V_1 V_2 V_3

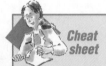

Precordial leads

The six unipolar precordial leads provide a view of the heart's horizontal plane and are placed in sequence across the chest.

Lead V_1
• Biphasic
• Distinguishes between right and left ventricular ectopic beats
• Monitors ventricular arrhythmias, ST-segment changes, and bundle-branch blocks

Leads V_2 and V_3
• Biphasic
• Used to detect ST-segment elevation

Lead V_4
• Produces a biphasic waveform

Lead V_5
• Produces a positive deflection on the ECG
• Can show changes in the ST segment or T wave (when used with V_4)

Lead V_6
• Produces a positive deflection on the ECG

In lead aV_R, the positive electrode is placed on the right arm (hence, the R) and produces a negative deflection because the heart's electrical activity moves away from the lead. In lead aV_L, the positive electrode is on the left arm and produces a positive deflection on the ECG. In lead aV_F, the positive electrode is on the left leg (despite the name aV_F) and produces a positive deflection.

These three limb leads also provide a view of the heart's frontal plane.

The preeminent precordials

The six unipolar precordial leads are placed in sequence across the chest and provide a view of the heart's horizontal plane. (See *Precordial views*.)

Lead V_1. The precordial lead V_1 electrode is placed on the right side of the sternum at the fourth intercostal rib space. This lead corresponds to the modified chest lead MCL_1 and shows the P wave, QRS complex, and ST segment particularly well. It helps to distinguish between right and left ventricular ectopic beats that result from myocardial irritation or other cardiac stimulation outside the normal conduction system. Lead V_1 is also useful in monitoring ventricular arrhythmias, ST-segment changes, and bundle-branch blocks.

Lead V_2. Lead V_2 is placed at the left of the sternum at the fourth intercostal rib space.

Lead V_3. Lead V_3 goes between V_2 and V_4. Leads V_1, V_2, and V_3 are biphasic, with both positive and negative deflections. Leads V_2 and V_3 can be used to detect ST-segment elevation.

Lead V_4. Lead V_4 is placed at the fifth intercostal space at the midclavicular line and produces a biphasic waveform.

Lead V_5. Lead V_5 is placed at the fifth intercostal space at the anterior axillary line. It produces a positive deflection on the ECG and, along with V_4, can show changes in the ST segment or T wave.

Lead V_6. Lead V_6, the last of the precordial leads is placed level with V_4 at the midaxillary line. Lead V_6 produces a positive deflection on the ECG.

The modest modified lead

Choose the lead MCL_1 to assess QRS-complex arrhythmias. The equivalent of the MCL_1 lead on the 12-lead ECG is V_1. MCL_1, is created by placing the negative electrode on the left upper chest, the positive electrode on the right side of the sternum at the fourth intercostal space, and the ground electrode usually on the right upper chest.

When the positive electrode is on the right side of the heart and the electrical current travels toward the left ventricle, the waveform has a negative deflection. As a result, ectopic or abnormal beats deflect in a positive direction.

You can use this lead to monitor premature ventricular beats and to distinguish different types of tachycardia, such as ventricular tachycardia and supraventricular tachycardia. Lead MCL_1 can

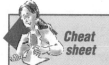

Cheat sheet

Modified leads

Lead MCL_1
• Equivalent of V_1
• Assesses QRS-complex arrhythmias, P-wave changes, and bundle-branch defects
• Monitors premature ventricular beats
• Distinguishes different types of tachycardia

Lead MCL_6
• Equivalent of V_6
• Monitors ventricular conduction changes

Leadwire systems

This chart shows the correct electrode positions for some of the leads you'll use most often — the five-leadwire, three-leadwire, and telemetry systems. The chart uses the abbreviations RA for the right arm, LA for the left arm, RL for the right leg, LL for the left leg, C for the chest, and G for the ground.

Electrode positions
In the three- and the five-leadwire systems, electrode positions for one lead may be identi-cal to those for another lead. When that happens, change the lead selector switch to the setting that corresponds to the lead you want. In some cases, you'll need to reposition the electrodes.

Telemetry
In a telemetry monitoring system, you can create the same leads as the other systems with just two electrodes and a ground wire.

Five-leadwire system	Three-leadwire system	Telemetry system

Lead I

Lead II

Lead III

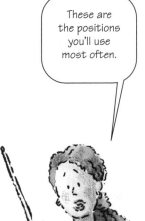

These are the positions you'll use most often.

Leadwire systems *(continued)*

Five-leadwire system	Three-leadwire system	Telemetry system

Lead MCL$_1$

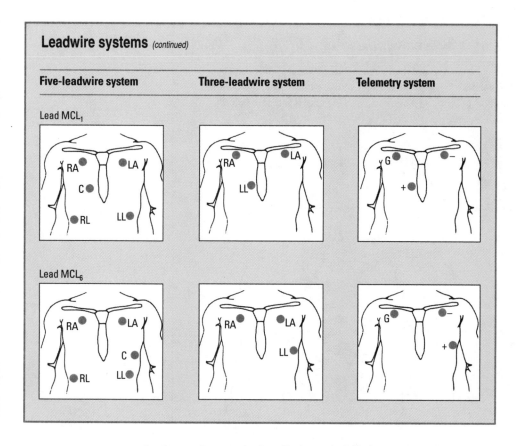

Lead MCL$_6$

also be used to assess bundle-branch defects and P-wave changes and to confirm pacemaker wire placement.

A positive option

MCL$_6$ monitors ventricular conduction changes. The positive lead in MCL$_6$ is placed in the same location as its equivalent, lead V$_6$. The positive electrode is placed at the fifth intercostal space at the midaxillary line, the negative electrode below the left shoulder, and the ground below the right shoulder.

Electrode basics

A three-, four-, or five-electrode system may be used for cardiac monitoring. (See *Leadwire systems.*) All three systems use a ground electrode to prevent accidental electrical shock to the patient.

Using a five-leadwire system

This illustration shows the correct placement of the leadwires for a five-leadwire system. The chest electrode shown is located in the V_1 position, but you can place it in any of the chest-lead positions. The electrodes are color-coded as follows.

- White—right arm (RA)
- Black—left arm (LA)
- Green—right leg (RL)

- Red—left leg (LL)
- Brown—chest (C)

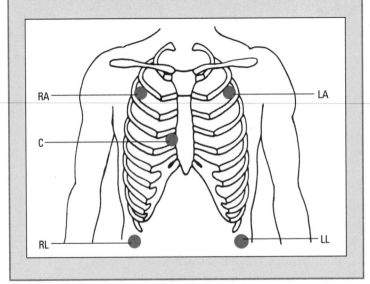

A three-electrode system has one positive electrode, one negative electrode, and a ground. A four-electrode system has a right leg electrode that becomes a permanent ground for all leads.

The popular five-electrode system is an extension of the four-electrode system and uses an additional exploratory chest lead to allow you to monitor any six modified chest leads as well as the standard limb leads. (See *Using a five-leadwire system.*) This system uses standardized chest placement. Wires that attach to the electrodes are usually color-coded to help you to place them correctly on the patient's chest.

How to apply electrodes

Before you attach electrodes to your patient, make sure he knows you're monitoring his heart rate and rhythm, not controlling them.

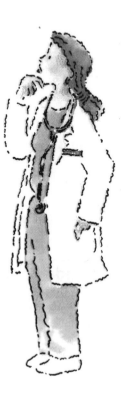

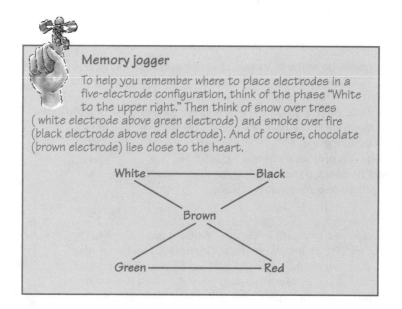

Memory jogger

To help you remember where to place electrodes in a five-electrode configuration, think of the phase "White to the upper right." Then think of snow over trees (white electrode above green electrode) and smoke over fire (black electrode above red electrode). And of course, chocolate (brown electrode) lies close to the heart.

White ———————— Black

Brown

Green ———————— Red

Tell him not to become upset if he hears an alarm during the procedure; it probably just means a leadwire has come loose.

Explain the electrode placement procedure to the patient, provide privacy, and wash your hands. Expose the patient's chest and select electrode sites for the chosen lead. Choose sites over soft tissues or close to bone, not over bony prominences, thick muscles, or skin folds. Those areas can produce ECG artifacts — waveforms not produced by the heart's electrical activity.

Prepare the skin

Next prepare the patient's skin. Use a special rough patch on the back of the electrode, a dry washcloth, or a gauze pad to briskly rub each site until the skin reddens. Be sure not to damage or break the skin. Brisk scrubbing helps to remove dead skin cells and improves electrical contact.

Care about hair

Hair may interfere with electrical contact. Therefore, clip dense hair closely at each site. Dry the areas if you moistened them.

If the patient has oily skin, clean each site with an alcohol pad and let it air-dry. This ensures proper adhesion and prevents the alcohol from becoming trapped beneath the electrode, which can irritate the skin and cause skin breakdown.

Stick it to me

To apply the electrodes, remove the backing and make sure each pregelled electrode is still moist. If an electrode has become dry, discard it and select another. A dry electrode decreases electrical contact and interferes with waveforms.

Apply one electrode to each prepared site using this method:
• Press one side of the electrode against the patient's skin, pull gently, and then press the opposite side of the electrode against the skin.
• Using two fingers, press the adhesive edge around the outside of the electrode to the patient's chest. This fixes the gel and stabilizes the electrode.
• Repeat this procedure for each electrode.
• Every 24 hours, remove the electrodes, assess the patient's skin, and put new electrodes in place.

Clip, clip, snap, snap

You'll also need to attach leadwires or cable connections to the monitor and attach leadwires to the electrodes. Leadwires may clip on or, more commonly, snap on. (See *Clip-on and snap-on leadwires.*) If you're using the snap-on type, attach the electrode to the leadwire before applying it to the patient's chest. You can even do this ahead of time if you know when the patient will arrive. Keep in mind that you may lose electrode contact if you press down to apply the leadwire.

When you use a clip-on leadwire, apply it after the electrode has been secured to the patient's skin. That way, applying the clip won't interfere with the electrode's contact with the skin.

Observing the cardiac rhythm

After the electrodes are in proper position, the monitor is on, and the necessary cables are attached, observe the screen. You should see the patient's ECG waveform. Although some monitoring systems allow you to make adjustments by touching the screen, most require you to manipulate knobs and buttons. If the waveform appears too large or too small, change the size by adjusting the gain control. If the waveform appears too high or too low on the screen, adjust the position dial.

Verify that the monitor detects each heartbeat by comparing the patient's apical rate with the rate displayed on the monitor. Set the upper and lower limits of the heart rate according to your facility's policy and the patient's condition. Heart rate alarms are generally set 10 to 20 beats per minute higher or lower than the patient's heart rate.

Monitors with arrhythmia detectors generate a rhythm strip automatically whenever the alarm goes off. You can obtain other views of your patient's cardiac rhythm by selecting different leads. You can select leads with the lead selector button or switch.

Clip-on and snap-on leadwires

Several kinds of leadwires are available for monitoring. A clip-on leadwire should be attached to the electrode *after* it has been placed on the patient's chest. A snap-on leadwire should be attached to the electrode *before* it has been placed on the patient's chest. Doing so prevents patient discomfort and disturbance of the contact between the electrode and the skin.

Clip-on leadwire

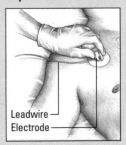

Leadwire
Electrode

Snap-on leadwire

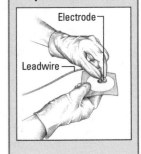

Electrode
Leadwire

Printing it out

To get a printout of the patient's cardiac rhythm, press the record control on the monitor. The ECG strip will be printed at the central console. Some systems print the rhythm from a recorder box on the monitor itself.

Most monitors allow you to input the date, time, and the patient's name and room number as a permanent record, but if the monitor you're using can't do this, label the rhythm strip with the date, time, patient's name, room number and rhythm interpretation. Add any appropriate clinical information to the ECG strip, such as any medication administered, presence of chest pain, or patient activity at the time of the recording. Be sure to place the rhythm strip in the appropriate section of the patient's medical record.

It's all on paper

Waveforms produced by the heart's electrical current are recorded on graphed ECG paper by a heated stylus. ECG paper consists of horizontal and vertical lines forming a grid. A piece of ECG paper is called an ECG strip or tracing. (See *ECG grid.*)

The horizontal axis of the ECG strip represents time. Each small block equals 0.04 second, and five small blocks form a large block, which equals 0.2 second. This time increment is determined by multiplying 0.04 second (for one small block) by 5, the number of small blocks that compose a large block. Five large blocks equal 1 second (5×0.2). When measuring or calculating a patient's heart rate, a 6-second strip consisting of 30 large blocks is usually used.

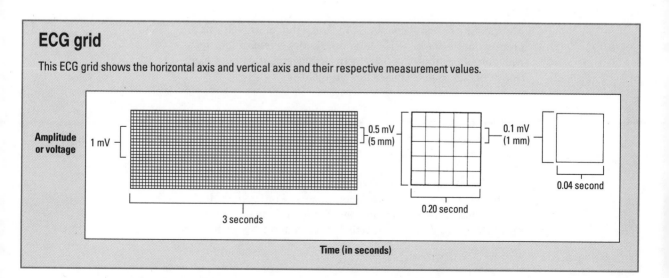

ECG grid

This ECG grid shows the horizontal axis and vertical axis and their respective measurement values.

Amplitude or voltage — 1 mV

0.5 mV (5 mm)

0.1 mV (1 mm)

0.04 second

3 seconds

0.20 second

Time (in seconds)

The ECG strip's vertical axis measures amplitude in millimeters (mm) or electrical voltage in millivolts (mV). Each small block represents 1 mm or 0.1 mV; each large block, 5 mm or 0.5 mV. To determine the amplitude of a wave, segment, or interval, count the number of small blocks from the baseline to the highest or lowest point of the wave, segment, or interval.

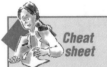

Cheat sheet

ECG strip

- 1 small horizontal block = 0.04 second
- 5 small horizontal blocks = 1 large block = 0.2 second
- 5 large horizontal blocks = 1 second
- Normal strip = 30 large horizontal blocks = 6 seconds
- 1 small vertical block = 0.1 mV
- 1 large vertical block = 0.5 mV
- Amplitude (mV) = number of small blocks from baseline to highest or lowest point

Troubleshooting problems

For optimal cardiac monitoring, you need to recognize problems that can interfere with obtaining a reliable ECG recording. (See *Troubleshooting monitor problems*.) Causes of interference include artifact from patient movement and poorly placed or poorly functioning equipment.

Artifact

Artifact, also called waveform interference, may be seen with excessive movement (somatic tremor). The baseline of the ECG appears wavy, bumpy, or tremulous. Dry electrodes may also cause this problem due to poor contact.

Interference

Electrical interference, also called 60-cycle interference, is caused by electrical power leakage. It may also occur due to interference from other room equipment or improperly grounded equipment. As a result, the lost current pulses at a rate of 60 cycles per second. This interference appears on the ECG as a baseline that's thick and unreadable.

Wandering baseline

A wandering baseline undulates, meaning that all waveforms are present but the baseline isn't stationary. Movement of the chest wall during respiration, poor electrode placement, or poor electrode contact usually causes this problem.

Faulty equipment

Faulty equipment, such as broken leadwires and cables, can also cause monitoring problems. Excessively worn equipment can cause improper grounding, putting the patient at risk for accidental shock.

Be aware that some types of artifact resemble arrhythmias, and the monitor will interpret them as such. For instance, the monitor may sense a small movement, such as the patient brushing his teeth, as a potentially lethal ventricular tachycardia. So re-

Mixed signals

Troubleshooting monitor problems

What you see	What might cause it	What to do about it
Artifact (waveform interference) 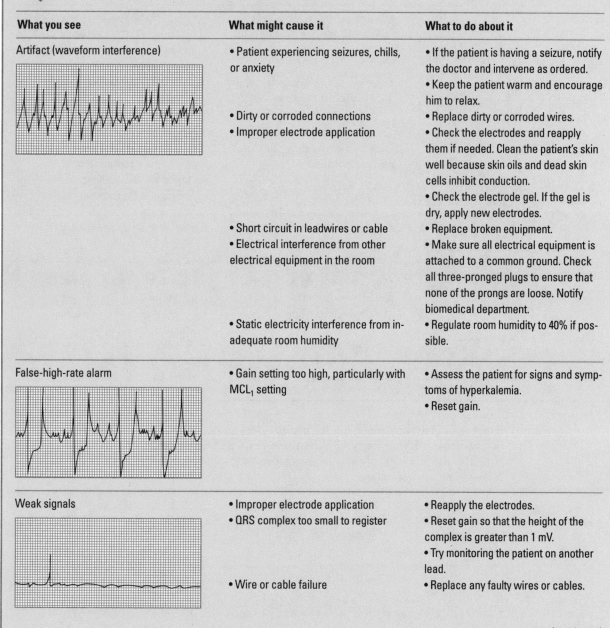	• Patient experiencing seizures, chills, or anxiety • Dirty or corroded connections • Improper electrode application • Short circuit in leadwires or cable • Electrical interference from other electrical equipment in the room • Static electricity interference from inadequate room humidity	• If the patient is having a seizure, notify the doctor and intervene as ordered. • Keep the patient warm and encourage him to relax. • Replace dirty or corroded wires. • Check the electrodes and reapply them if needed. Clean the patient's skin well because skin oils and dead skin cells inhibit conduction. • Check the electrode gel. If the gel is dry, apply new electrodes. • Replace broken equipment. • Make sure all electrical equipment is attached to a common ground. Check all three-pronged plugs to ensure that none of the prongs are loose. Notify biomedical department. • Regulate room humidity to 40% if possible.
False-high-rate alarm	• Gain setting too high, particularly with MCL_1 setting	• Assess the patient for signs and symptoms of hyperkalemia. • Reset gain.
Weak signals	• Improper electrode application • QRS complex too small to register • Wire or cable failure	• Reapply the electrodes. • Reset gain so that the height of the complex is greater than 1 mV. • Try monitoring the patient on another lead. • Replace any faulty wires or cables.

(continued)

Troubleshooting monitor problems *(continued)*

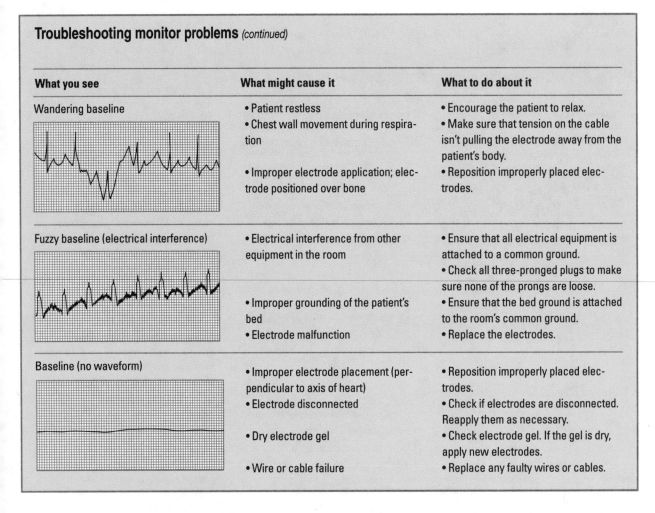

What you see	What might cause it	What to do about it
Wandering baseline	• Patient restless • Chest wall movement during respiration • Improper electrode application; electrode positioned over bone	• Encourage the patient to relax. • Make sure that tension on the cable isn't pulling the electrode away from the patient's body. • Reposition improperly placed electrodes.
Fuzzy baseline (electrical interference)	• Electrical interference from other equipment in the room • Improper grounding of the patient's bed • Electrode malfunction	• Ensure that all electrical equipment is attached to a common ground. • Check all three-pronged plugs to make sure none of the prongs are loose. • Ensure that the bed ground is attached to the room's common ground. • Replace the electrodes.
Baseline (no waveform)	• Improper electrode placement (perpendicular to axis of heart) • Electrode disconnected • Dry electrode gel • Wire or cable failure	• Reposition improperly placed electrodes. • Check if electrodes are disconnected. Reapply them as necessary. • Check electrode gel. If the gel is dry, apply new electrodes. • Replace any faulty wires or cables.

member to treat the patient, not the monitor. The more familiar you become with your unit's monitoring system—and with your patient—the more quickly you can recognize and interpret problems and act appropriately.

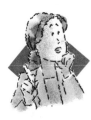

Quick quiz

1. On ECG graph paper, the horizontal axis measures:
   A. time.
   B. speed.
   C. voltage.

Answer: A. The horizontal axis measures time and is recorded in increments of 0.04 second for each small box.

2. On ECG graph paper, the vertical axis measures:
   A. time.
   B. speed.
   C. voltage.

Answer: C. The vertical axis measures voltage by the height of a waveform.

3. The leads not included in a 12-lead ECG are:
   A. II and III.
   B. V_1 and V_3.
   C. MCL_1 and MCL_6.

Answer: C. The modified chest leads MCL_1 and MCL_6 are equivalent to leads V_1 and V_6 of the 12-lead ECG, but they're actually bipolar limb leads and aren't included in a 12-lead ECG.

4. A biphasic deflection will occur on an ECG if the electrical current is traveling in a direction:
   A. posterior to the positive electrode.
   B. perpendicular to the positive electrode.
   C. superior to the positive electrode.

Answer: B. A current traveling in a route perpendicular to the positive electrode will generate a biphasic wave, partially above and below the isoelectric line.

5. If a lead comes off the patient's chest, the waveform:
   A. will appear much larger on the monitor.
   B. will appear much smaller on the monitor.
   C. won't be seen at all on the monitor.

Answer: C. Leadwire disconnection will stop the monitoring process, and the waveform won't be seen on the monitor.

6.   To monitor lead II, you would place the:
A.   positive electrode below the lowest palpable rib at the left midclavicular line and the negative electrode below the right clavicle.
B.   positive electrode below the right clavicle at the midline and the negative electrode below the left clavicle at the midline.
C.   positive electrode below the left clavicle and the negative electrode below the right clavicle at the midclavicular line.

Answer: A. This electrode position is the proper one for monitoring in lead II.

Scoring

☆☆☆   If you answered all six questions correctly, superb! We're ready to go out on a limb lead for you!

☆☆   If you answered four or five questions correctly, great! We hardly need to monitor your progress!

☆   If you answered fewer than four questions correctly, keep at it! We like the way your current flows!

3

Interpreting a rhythm strip

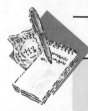

Just the facts

This chapter explains how the ECG represents electrical impulses as they travel through the heart. In this chapter, you'll learn:

♦ about the components of an ECG complex as well as their significance and variations

♦ how to calculate the rate and rhythm of an ECG recording

♦ the step-by-step approach to ECG interpretation

♦ how to identify normal sinus rhythm.

A look at an ECG complex

An electrocardiogram (ECG) complex represents the electrical events occurring in one cardiac cycle. A complex consists of five waveforms labeled with the letters P, Q, R, S, and T. The middle three letters — Q, R, and S — are referred to as a unit, the QRS complex. ECG tracings represent the conduction of electrical impulses from the atria to the ventricles. (See *Normal ECG*, page 46.)

The P wave

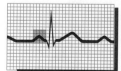

The P wave is the first component of a normal ECG waveform. It represents atrial depolarization — conduction of an electrical impulse through the atria. When evaluating a P wave, look closely at its characteristics, especially its location, configuration, and deflection. A normal P wave has the following characteristics:

• location — precedes the QRS complex
• amplitude — 2 to 3 mm high
• duration — 0.06 to 0.12 second
• configuration — usually rounded and upright

• deflection—positive or upright in leads I, II, aV$_F$, and V$_2$ to V$_6$; usually positive but variable in leads III and aV$_L$; negative or inverted in lead aV$_R$; biphasic or variable in lead V$_1$.

If the deflection and configuration of a P wave are normal—for example, if the P wave is upright in lead II and is rounded and smooth—and if the P wave precedes each QRS complex, you can assume that this electrical impulse originated in the sinoatrial (SA) node. The atria start to contract partway through the P wave,

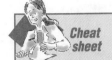

Normal P wave

• *Location*—precedes the QRS complex
• *Amplitude*—2 to 3 mm high
• *Duration* — 0.06 to 0.12 second
• *Configuration*—usually rounded and upright
• *Deflection* — positive or upright in leads I, II, aV$_F$, and V$_2$ to V$_6$; usually positive but may vary in leads III and aV$_L$; negative or inverted in lead aV$_R$; biphasic or variable in lead V$_1$

Normal ECG

This strip shows the components of a normal ECG waveform.

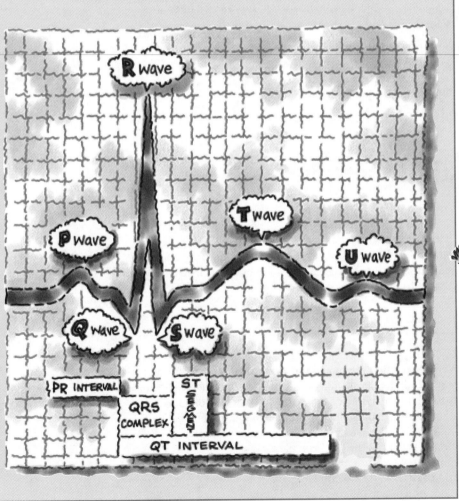

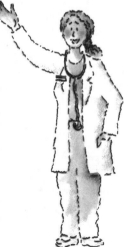

but you won't see this on the ECG. Remember, the ECG records electrical activity only, not mechanical activity or contraction.

The odd Ps

Peaked, notched, or enlarged P waves may represent atrial hypertrophy or enlargement associated with chronic obstructive pulmonary disease, pulmonary emboli, valvular disease, or heart failure. Inverted P waves may signify retrograde or reverse conduction from the atrioventricular (AV) junction toward the atria. When an upright sinus P wave becomes inverted, consider retrograde or reverse conduction as possible conditions.

Varying P waves indicate that the impulse may be coming from different sites, as with a wandering pacemaker rhythm, irritable atrial tissue, or damage near the SA node. Absent P waves may signify conduction by a route other than the SA node, as with a junctional or atrial fibrillation rhythm.

The PR interval

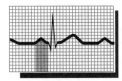

The PR interval tracks the atrial impulse from the atria through the AV node, bundle of His, and right and left bundle branches. When evaluating a PR interval, look especially at its duration. Changes in the PR interval indicate an altered impulse formation or a conduction delay, as seen in AV block. A normal PR interval has the following characteristics (amplitude, configuration, and deflection aren't measured):
• location—from the beginning of the P wave to the beginning of the QRS complex
• duration—0.12 to 0.20 second.

The short and long of it

Short PR intervals (less than 0.12 second) indicate that the impulse originated somewhere other than the SA node. This variation is associated with junctional arrhythmias and preexcitation syndromes. Prolonged PR intervals (greater than 0.20 second) may represent a conduction delay through the atria or AV junction due to digoxin toxicity or heart block—slowing related to ischemia or conduction tissue disease.

The QRS complex

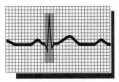

The QRS complex follows the P wave and represents depolarization of the ventricles, or impulse conduction. Immediately after the ventricles depolarize, as represented by the QRS complex,

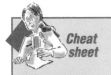

Cheat sheet

Normal PR interval

• *Location*—from the beginning of the P wave to the beginning of the QRS complex
• *Duration*—0.12 to 0.20 second

QRS waveform variety

The illustrations below show the various configurations of QRS complexes. When documenting the QRS complex, use uppercase letters to indicate a wave with a normal or high amplitude (greater than 5 mm) and lowercase letters to indicate a wave with a low amplitude (less than 5 mm).

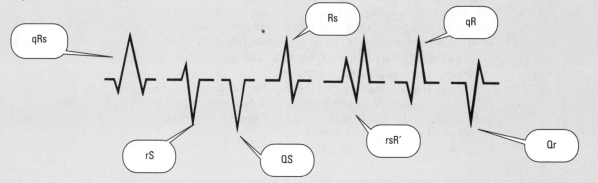

they contract. That contraction ejects blood from the ventricles and pumps it through the arteries, creating a pulse.

Not necessarily mechanical

Whenever you're monitoring cardiac rhythm, remember that the waveform you see represents the heart's electrical activity only. It doesn't guarantee a mechanical contraction of the heart and a subsequent pulse. The contraction could be weak, as happens with premature ventricular contractions, or absent, as happens with pulseless electrical activity. So before you treat the strip, check the patient.

It's all normal

Pay special attention to the duration and configuration when evaluating a QRS complex. A normal complex has the following characteristics:
- location—follows the PR interval
- amplitude—5 to 30 mm high but differs for each lead used
- duration—0.06 to 0.10 second, or half of the PR interval. Duration is measured from the beginning of the Q wave to the end of the S wave or from the beginning of the R wave if the Q wave is absent.
- configuration—consists of the Q wave (the first negative deflection, or deflection above the baseline, after the P wave), the R wave (the first positive deflection after the Q wave), and the S wave (the first negative deflection after the R wave). You may not always see all three waves. The ventricles depolarize quickly,

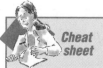

Cheat sheet

Normal QRS complex

- *Location* — follows the PR interval
- Amplitude—5 to 30 mm high but differs for each lead used
- *Duration*—0.06 to 0.10 second, or half the PR interval
- *Configuration* — consists of the Q wave, the R wave, and the S wave
- *Deflection* — positive in leads I, II, III, aV$_L$, aV$_F$, and V$_4$ to V$_6$ and negative in leads aV$_R$ and V$_1$ to V$_3$

minimizing contact time between the stylus and the ECG paper, so the QRS complex typically appears thinner than other ECG components. It may also look different in each lead. (See *QRS waveform variety.*)
• deflection—positive in leads I, II, III, aV_L, aV_F, and V_4 to V_6 and negative in leads aV_R and V_1 to V_3.

Crucial I.D.

Remember that the QRS complex represents intraventricular conduction time. That's why identifying and correctly interpreting it is so crucial. If no P wave appears with the QRS complex, then the impulse may have originated in the ventricles, indicating a ventricular arrhythmia.

Deep and wide

Deep, wide Q waves may represent myocardial infarction. In this case, the Q-wave amplitude is 25% of the R-wave amplitude, or the duration of the Q wave is 0.04 second or more. A notched R wave may signify a bundle-branch block. A widened QRS complex (greater than 0.12 second) may signify a ventricular conduction delay. A missing QRS complex may indicate AV block or ventricular standstill.

The ST segment

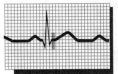

The ST segment represents the end of ventricular conduction or depolarization and the beginning of ventricular recovery or repolarization. The point that marks the end of the QRS complex and the beginning of the ST segment is known as the J point.

Normal ST

Pay special attention to the deflection of an ST segment. A normal ST segment has the following characteristics (amplitude, duration, and configuration aren't observed):
• location—extends from the S wave to the beginning of the T wave
• deflection—usually isoelectric (neither positive nor negative); may vary from –0.5 to +1 mm in some precordial leads.

Not so normal ST

A change in the ST segment may indicate myocardial damage. An ST segment may become either elevated or depressed. (See *Changes in the ST segment,* page 50.)

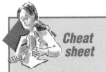

Cheat sheet

Normal ST segment

• *Location*—from the S wave to the beginning of the T wave
• *Deflection*—usually isoelectric; may vary from –0.5 to +1 mm in some precordial leads

Changes in the ST segment

Closely monitoring the ST segment on a patient's ECG can help you detect ischemia or injury before infarction develops.

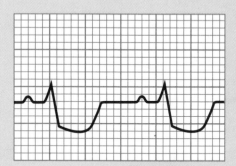

ST-segment depression

An ST segment is considered depressed when it's 0.5 mm or more below the baseline. A depressed ST segment may indicate myocardial ischemia or digoxin toxicity.

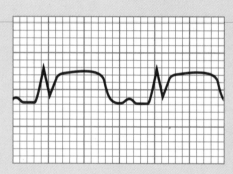

ST-segment elevation

An ST segment is considered elevated when it's 1 mm or more above the baseline. An elevated ST segment may indicate myocardial injury.

The T wave

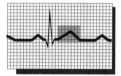

The T wave represents ventricular recovery or repolarization. When evaluating a T wave, look at the amplitude, configuration, and deflection. Normal T waves have the following characteristics (duration isn't measured):

- location—follows the S wave
- amplitude—0.5 mm in leads I, II, and III and up to 10 mm in the precordial leads
- configuration—typically round and smooth
- deflection—usually upright in leads I, II, and V_3 to V_6; inverted in lead aV_R; variable in all other leads.

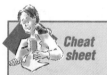

Cheat sheet

Normal T wave

- *Location*—follows the S wave
- *Amplitude*—0.5 mm in leads I, II, and III and up to 10 mm in the precordial leads
- *Configuration*—typically round and smooth
- *Deflection*—usually upright in leads I, II, and V_3 to V_6; inverted in lead aV_R; variable in all other leads

Why is that T so bumpy?

The T wave's peak represents the relative refractory period of ventricular repolarization, a period during which cells are especially vulnerable to extra stimuli. Bumps in a T wave may indicate that a P wave is hidden in it. If a P wave is hidden, atrial depolarization has occurred, the impulse having originated at a site above the ventricles.

Tall, inverted, or pointy Ts

Tall, peaked, or tented T waves indicate myocardial injury or hyperkalemia. Inverted T waves in leads I, II, or V_3 through V_6 may represent myocardial ischemia. Heavily notched or pointed T waves in an adult may mean pericarditis.

The QT interval

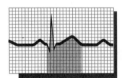

The QT interval measures ventricular depolarization and repolarization. The length of the QT interval varies according to heart rate. The faster the heart rate, the shorter the QT interval. When checking the QT interval, look closely at the duration.

A normal QT interval has the following characteristics (amplitude, configuration, and deflection aren't observed):
• location—extends from the beginning of the QRS complex to the end of the T wave
• duration—varies according to age, sex, and heart rate; usually lasts from 0.36 to 0.44 second; shouldn't be greater than half the distance between consecutive R waves when the rhythm is regular.

The importance of QT

The QT interval shows the time needed for the ventricular depolarization-repolarization cycle. An abnormality in duration may indicate myocardial problems. Prolonged QT intervals indicate prolonged ventricular repolarization, meaning that the relative refractory period is longer.

This variation is also associated with certain medications such as type I antiarrhythmics. Prolonged QT syndrome is a congenital conduction-system defect present in certain families. Short QT intervals may result from digoxin toxicity or hypercalcemia.

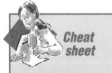

Cheat sheet

Normal QT interval

• *Location*—from the beginning of the QRS complex to the end of the T wave
• *Duration*—varies; usually lasts from 0.36 to 0.44 second

The U wave

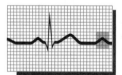

The U wave represents the recovery period of the Purkinje or ventricular conduction fibers. It isn't present on every rhythm strip. The configuration is the most important characteristic of the U wave.

When present, a normal U wave has the following characteristics (amplitude and duration aren't measured):

- location—follows the T wave
- configuration—typically upright and rounded
- deflection—upright.

The U wave may not appear on an ECG. A prominent U wave may be due to hypercalcemia, hypokalemia, or digoxin toxicity.

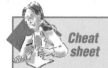

Cheat sheet

Normal U wave

- *Location*—follows T wave
- *Configuration*—typically upright and rounded
- *Deflection*—upright

8-step method

Interpreting a rhythm strip is a skill developed through practice. You can use several methods, as long as you're consistent. (See *Methods of measuring rhythm.*) Rhythm strip analysis requires a sequential and systematic approach such as that which employs the eight steps outlined here.

Step 1: Determine the rhythm.

To determine the heart's atrial and ventricular rhythms, use either the paper-and-pencil method or the caliper method.

For atrial rhythm, measure the P-P intervals—the intervals between consecutive P waves. These intervals should occur regularly with only small variations associated with respirations. Then compare the P-P intervals in several cycles. Consistently similar P-P intervals indicate regular atrial rhythm; dissimilar P-P intervals indicate irregular atrial rhythm.

To determine the ventricular rhythm, measure the intervals between two consecutive R waves in the QRS complexes. If an R wave isn't present, use either the Q wave or the S wave of consecutive QRS complexes. The R-R intervals should occur regularly.

Then compare R-R intervals in several cycles. As with atrial rhythms, consistently similar intervals mean a regular rhythm; dissimilar intervals point to an irregular rhythm.

Ask yourself: How irregular is the rhythm? Is it slightly irregular or markedly so? Does the irregularity occur in a pattern (a regularly irregular pattern)? Keep in mind that variations of up to 0.04 second are considered normal.

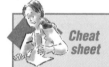

Cheat sheet

8-step method

- Step 1: Determine the rhythm.
- Step 2: Determine the rate.
- Step 3: Evaluate the P wave.
- Step 4: Measure the PR interval.
- Step 5: Determine the QRS duration.
- Step 6: Examine the T waves.
- Step 7: Measure the QT interval.
- Step 8: Check for ectopic beats and other abnormalities.

Methods of measuring rhythm

You can use either of the following methods to determine atrial or ventricular rhythm.

Paper-and-pencil method

Place the ECG strip on a flat surface. Then position the straight edge of a piece of paper along the strip's baseline. Move the paper up slightly so the straight edge is near the peak of the R wave.

With a pencil, mark the paper at the R waves of two consecutive QRS complexes, as shown at right. This is the R-R interval. Next, move the paper across the strip, aligning the two marks with succeeding R-R intervals. If the distance for each R-R interval is the same, the ventricular rhythm is regular. If the distance varies, the rhythm is irregular.

Use the same method to measure the distance between the P waves (the P-P interval) and determine whether the atrial rhythm is regular or irregular.

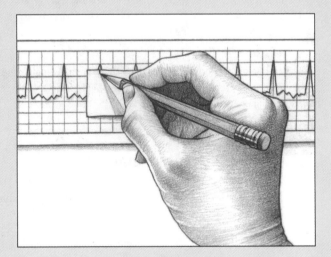

Caliper method

With the ECG on a flat surface, place one point of the caliper on the peak of the first R wave of two consecutive QRS complexes. Then adjust the caliper legs so the other point is on the peak of the next R wave, as shown at right. This distance is the R-R interval.

Now pivot the first point of the caliper toward the third R wave and note whether it falls on the peak of that wave. Check succeeding R-R intervals in the same way. If they're all the same, the ventricular rhythm is regular. If they vary, the rhythm is irregular.

Using the same method, measure the P-P intervals to determine whether the atrial rhythm is regular or irregular.

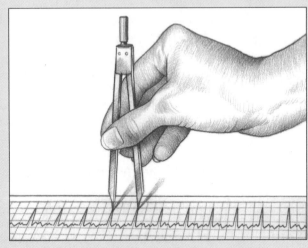

Step 2: Determine the rate.

You can use one of three methods to determine atrial and ventricular heart rate. Remember, don't rely on those methods alone. Always check a pulse to correlate it with the heart rate on the ECG.

Calculating the heart rate

This table can help make the sequencing method of determining heart rate more precise. After counting the number of boxes between the R waves, use this table to find the rate.

For example, if you count 20 small blocks or 4 large blocks, the rate would be 75 beats/minute. To calculate the atrial rate, use the same method with P waves instead of R waves.

Rapid estimation

This rapid-rate calculation is also called the countdown method. Using the number of large boxes between R waves or P waves as a guide, you can rapidly estimate ventricular or atrial rates by memorizing the sequence "300, 150, 100, 75, 60, 50."

Number of small blocks	Heart rate
5 (1 large block)	300
6	250
7	214
8	187
9	166
10 (2 large blocks)	150
11	136
12	125
13	115
14	107
15 (3 large blocks)	100
16	94
17	88
18	83
19	79
20 (4 large blocks)	75
21	71
22	68
23	65
24	63
25 (5 large blocks)	60
26	58
27	56
28	54
29	52
30 (6 large blocks)	50
31	48
32	47
33	45
34	44
35 (7 large blocks)	43
36	41
37	40
38	39
39	38
40 (8 large blocks)	37

10-times method

The easiest way to calculate rate is the 10-times method, especially if the rhythm is irregular. You'll notice that ECG paper is marked in increments of 3 seconds, or 15 large boxes. To figure the atrial rate, obtain a 6-second strip, count the number of P waves, and multiply by 10. Ten 6-second strips represent 1 minute. Calculate ventricular rate the same way, using the R waves.

1,500 method

If the heart rhythm is regular, use the 1,500 method, so named because 1,500 small squares represent 1 minute. Count the small squares between identical points on two consecutive P waves and then divide 1,500 by that number to get the atrial rate. To obtain the ventricular rate, use the same method with two consecutive R waves.

Sequence method

The third method of estimating heart rate is the sequence method, which requires that you memorize a sequence of numbers. (See *Calculating the heart rate*.) To get the atrial rate, find a P wave that peaks on a heavy black line and assign the following numbers to the next six heavy black lines: 300, 150, 100, 75, 60, and 50. Then find the next P wave peak and estimate the atrial rate, based on the number assigned to the nearest heavy black line. Estimate the ventricular rate the same way, using the R wave.

Where P waves should be

In this 6-second rhythm strip, each P wave is followed by a QRS complex, as it normally would be.

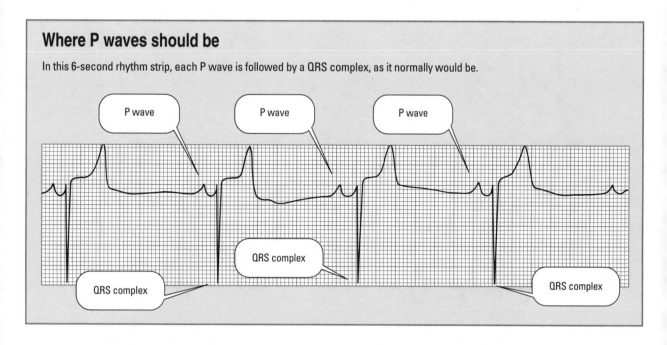

Step 3: Evaluate the P wave.

When examining a rhythm strip for P waves, ask yourself: Are P waves present? Do they all have normal configurations? Do they all have a similar size and shape? Does every P wave have a QRS complex? (See *Where P waves should be*.)

Step 4: Determine the duration of the PR interval.

To measure the PR interval, count the small squares between the start of the P wave and the start of the QRS complex; then multiply the number of squares by 0.04 second. Now ask yourself: Is the duration a normal 0.12 to 0.20 second? Is the PR interval constant?

Step 5: Determine the duration of the QRS complex.

When determining QRS duration, be sure to measure straight across from the end of the PR interval to the end of the S wave, not just to the peak. Remember, the QRS has no horizontal components. To calculate duration, count the number of small squares between the beginning and end of the QRS complex and multiply this number by 0.04 second. Then ask yourself: Is the duration a normal 0.06 to 0.10 second? Are all QRS complexes the same size

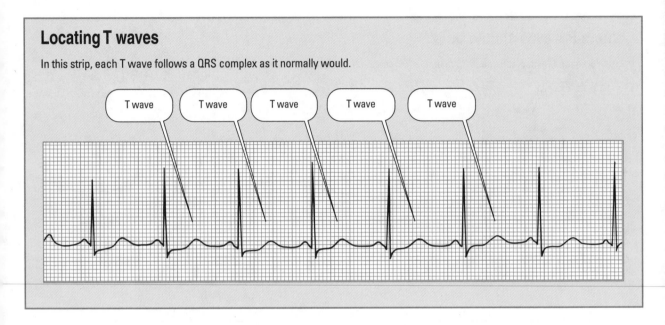

Locating T waves

In this strip, each T wave follows a QRS complex as it normally would.

T wave   T wave   T wave   T wave   T wave

and shape? (If not, measure each one and describe it individually.)
Does a QRS complex appear after every P wave?

Step 6: Evaluate the T waves.

Examine the strip for T waves. Then ask yourself: Are T waves
present? Do they all have a normal shape? Do they all have a normal amplitude? Do they all have the same amplitude as the QRS
complexes? (See *Locating T waves*.)

Step 7: Determine the duration of the QT interval.

Count the number of small squares between the beginning of the
QRS complex and the end of the T wave, where the T wave returns to the baseline. Multiply this number by 0.04 second. Ask
yourself: Is the duration a normal 0.36 to 0.44 second?

Step 8: Evaluate any other components.

Check for ectopic beats and other abnormalities. Also check the
ST segment for abnormalities, and look for the presence of a
U wave. Note your findings, and then interpret them by naming
the rhythm strip according to one or all of these findings:

- origin of the rhythm (for example, sinus node, atria, AV node, or ventricles)
- rate characteristics (for example, bradycardia or tachycardia)
- rhythm abnormalities (for example, flutter, fibrillation, heart block, escape rhythm, or other arrhythmias).

Recognizing normal sinus rhythm

Before you can recognize an arrhythmia, you first need to be able to recognize normal sinus rhythm. Normal sinus rhythm records an impulse that starts in the sinus node and progresses to the ventricles through a normal conduction pathway—from the sinus node to the atria and AV node, through the bundle of His, to the bundle branches, and on to the Purkinje fibers. Normal sinus rhythm is the standard against which all other rhythms are compared. (See *Normal sinus rhythm.*)

Normal sinus rhythm

Normal sinus rhythm, shown below, represents normal impulse conduction through the heart.

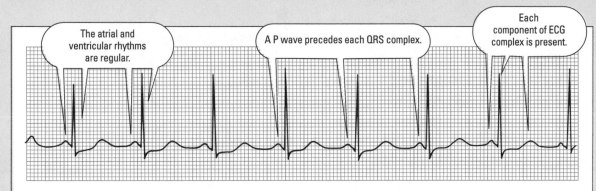

Characteristics of normal sinus rhythm include:

- regular rhythm
- normal rate
- a P wave for every QRS complex; all P waves similar in size and shape
- all QRS complexes similar in size and shape
- normal PR and QT intervals
- normal (upright and round) T waves.

What makes for normal?

Using the 8-step method previously described, these are the characteristics of normal sinus rhythm:
• Atrial and ventricular rhythms are regular.
• Atrial and ventricular rates fall between 60 and 100 beats/minute, the SA node's normal firing rate, and all impulses are conducted to the ventricles.
• P waves are rounded, smooth, and upright in lead II, signaling that a sinus impulse has reached the atria.
• The PR interval is normal (0.12 to 0.20 second), indicating that the impulse is following normal conduction pathways.
• The QRS complex is of normal duration (less than 0.12 second), representing normal ventricular impulse conduction and recovery.
• The T wave is upright in lead II, confirming that normal repolarization has taken place.
• The QT interval is within normal limits (0.36 to 0.44 second).
• No ectopic or aberrant beats are occurring.

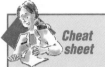

Cheat sheet

Normal sinus rhythm

This is the standard against which all other rhythms are compared.

Characteristics
• Regular rhythm
• Normal rate
• P wave for every QRS complex; all P waves similar in size and shape
• All QRS complexes similar in size and shape
• Normal PR and QT intervals
• Normal T waves

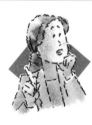

Quick quiz

1. The P wave represents:
   A. atrial repolarization.
   B. atrial depolarization.
   C. ventricular depolarization.

   Answer: B. The impulse spreading across the atria generates a P wave.

2. The normal duration of a QRS complex is:
   A. 0.06 to 0.10 second.
   B. 0.12 to 0.20 second.
   C. 0.36 to 0.44 second.

   Answer: A. This time frame—0.06 to 0.10 second—represents ventricular depolarization.

3. To gather information about impulse conduction from the atria to the ventricles, study the:
   A. P wave.
   B. PR interval.
   C. ST segment.

   Answer: B. The PR interval measures the interval between atrial depolarization and ventricular depolarization. A normal PR interval is 0.12 to 0.20 second.

4. The period when myocardial cells are vulnerable to extra stimuli begins with the:
- A.   end of the P wave.
- B.   start of the R wave.
- C.   peak of the T wave.

Answer: C. The peak of the T wave represents the beginning of the relative, although not the absolute, refractory period, when the cells are vulnerable to stimuli.

5. Atrial and ventricular rates can be determined by counting the number of small boxes between:
- A.   the end of one P wave and the beginning of another.
- B.   two consecutive P or R waves.
- C.   the middle of two consecutive T waves.

Answer: B. Atrial and ventricular rates can be determined by counting the number of small boxes between two consecutive P or R waves and then dividing that number into 1,500.

Test strips

Now try these test strips. Fill in the blanks below with the particular characteristics of the strip.

Strip 1

Atrial rhythm: _____   QRS complex: _____
Ventricular rhythm: _____   T wave:_____
Atrial rate: _____   QT interval: _____
Ventricular rate: _____   Other: _____
P wave:_____   **Interpretation:** _____
PR interval: _____

Strip 2

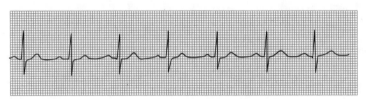

Atrial rhythm: _____   QRS complex: _____
Ventricular rhythm: _____   T wave: _____
Atrial rate: _____   QT interval: _____
Ventricular rate: _____   Other: _____
P wave: _____   **Interpretation:** _____
PR interval: _____

Answers to test strips

1. Rhythm: both atrial and ventricular rhythms are regular
Rate: atrial and ventricular rates are both 79 beats/minute
P wave: normal size and configuration
PR interval: 0.12 second
QRS complex: 0.08 second; normal size and configuration
T wave: normal configuration
QT interval: 0.44 second
Other: none
Interpretation: normal sinus rhythm

2. Rhythm: both atrial and ventricular rhythms are regular
Rate: atrial and ventricular rates are both 72 beats/minute
P wave: normal size and configuration
PR interval: 0.20 second
QRS complex: 0.10 second; normal size and configuration
T wave: normal configuration
QT interval: 0.42 second
Other: none
Interpretation: normal sinus rhythm

Scoring

☆☆☆   If you answered all seven questions correctly and filled in all the blanks pretty much as we did, hooray! You can read our rhythm strips anytime!

☆☆   If you answered five or six questions correctly and filled in most of the blanks the way we did, excellent! You deserve a shiny new pair of calipers!

☆   If you answered fewer than five questions correctly and missed most of the blanks, chin up! You're still tops with us!

Part II

Recognizing arrhythmias

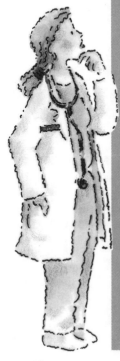

Sinus node arrhythmias

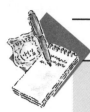

Just the facts

This chapter will help you identify the various sinus node arrhythmias—sinus arrhythmia, sinus bradycardia, sinus tachycardia, sinus arrest, and sick sinus syndrome. In this chapter, you'll learn:

♦ what role the sinoatrial (SA) node plays in arrhythmia formation

♦ which arrhythmias are generated from the SA node

♦ the cause, significance, treatment, and nursing implications of each arrhythmia

♦ which assessment findings are associated with each arrhythmia

♦ how to correctly interpret sinus node arrhythmias on an electrocardiogram.

A look at sinus node arrhythmias

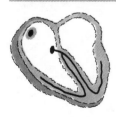

When the heart functions normally, the sinoatrial (SA) node, also called the sinus node, acts as the primary pacemaker. The sinus node assumes this role because its automatic firing rate exceeds that of the heart's other pacemakers. In an adult at rest, the sinus node has an inherent firing rate of 60 to 100 times/minute.

The SA node's blood supply comes from the right coronary artery and left circumflex artery. The autonomic nervous system richly innervates the sinus node through the vagal nerve, a parasympathetic nerve, and several sympathetic nerves. Stimulation of the vagus nerve decreases the node's firing rate, and stimulation of the sympathetic system increases it.

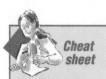

Cheat sheet

SA node

• Acts as primary pacemaker
• Inherent firing rate of 60 to 100 times/minute in a resting adult
• Supplied by blood from the right coronary artery and left circumflex artery

Sinus arrhythmia

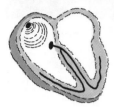

In sinus arrhythmia, the pacemaker cells of the SA node fire irregularly. The cardiac rate stays within normal limits, but the rhythm is irregular and corresponds to the respiratory cycle. Sinus arrhythmia can occur naturally in athletes, children, and older adults, but it rarely occurs in infants. Conditions unrelated to respiration may also produce sinus arrhythmia, including inferior-wall myocardial infarction (MI), advanced age, use of digoxin or morphine, and conditions involving increased intracranial pressure.

How it happens

Sinus arrhythmia, the heart's normal response to respirations, results from an inhibition of reflex vagal activity, or tone. During inspiration, an increase in the flow of blood back to the heart reduces vagal tone, which increases the heart rate. Electrocardiogram (ECG) complexes fall closer together, which shortens the P-P interval, the time elapsed between two consecutive P waves.

During expiration, venous return decreases, which in turn increases vagal tone, slows the heart rate, and lengthens the P-P interval. (See *Breathing and sinus arrhythmia*.)

Breathing and sinus arrhythmia

When sinus arrhythmia is related to respirations, you'll see an increase in heart rate with inspiration and a decrease with expiration, as shown here.

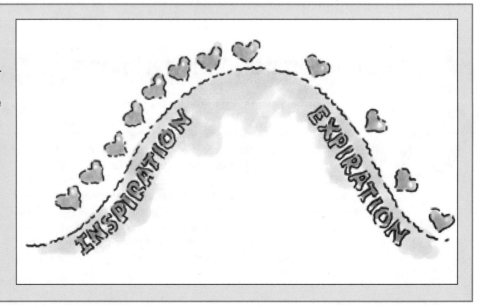

Sick sinus

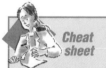

Sinus arrhythmia usually isn't significant and produces no symptoms. A marked variation in P-P intervals in an older adult, however, may indicate sick sinus syndrome, a related, potentially more serious phenomenon.

What to look for

When you look for sinus arrhythmia, you'll see that the rhythm is irregular and corresponds to the respiratory cycle. (See *Recognizing sinus arrhythmia.*) The difference between the shortest and longest P-P intervals — and the shortest and longest R-R intervals — exceeds 0.12 second.

The atrial and ventricular rates are within normal limits (60 to 100 beats/minute) and vary with respiration — faster with inspiration, slower with expiration. All other parameters are normal, except for the QT interval, which may vary slightly but remains normal.

It's all in the breath

Look for a peripheral pulse rate that increases during inspiration and decreases during expiration. If the arrhythmia is caused by an underlying condition, you may note signs and symptoms of that condition.

Cheat sheet

Indicators of sinus arrhythmia

• *Rhythm*—irregular, corresponding to the respiratory cycle
• *Atrial and ventricular rates*—within normal limits; vary with respiration
• *Other parameters*— QT interval may vary slightly

Recognizing sinus arrhythmia

The following rhythm strip illustrates sinus arrhythmia. Look for these distinguishing characteristics:

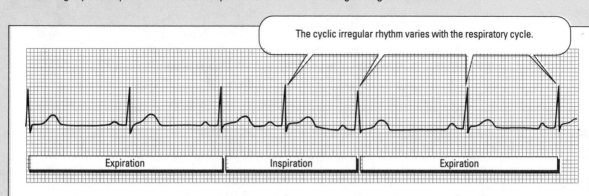

The cyclic irregular rhythm varies with the respiratory cycle.

Expiration | Inspiration | Expiration

• *Rhythm:* irregular
• *Rate:* 60 beats/minute
• *P wave:* normal

• *PR interval:* 0.16 second
• *QRS complex:* 0.06 second
• *T wave:* normal

• *QT interval:* 0.36 second
• *Other:* phasic slowing and quickening.

Mixed signals

A longer look at sinus arrhythmia

Don't mistake sinus arrhythmia for other rhythms. At first glance it may look like atrial fibrillation, normal sinus rhythm with premature atrial contractions, sinoatrial block, or sinus pauses. Observe the monitor and the patient's respiratory pattern for several minutes to determine the rate and rhythm. And, as always, check the patient's pulse.

Sinus arrhythmia is easier to detect when the heart rate is slow; it may disappear when the heart rate increases, as with exercise or after atropine administration.

How you intervene

Unless the patient is symptomatic, treatment usually isn't necessary. If sinus arrhythmia is unrelated to respirations, the underlying cause may require treatment.

When caring for a patient with sinus arrhythmia, observe the heart rhythm during respiration to determine whether the arrhythmia coincides with the respiratory cycle. Be sure to check the monitor carefully to avoid an inaccurate interpretation of the waveform. (See *A longer look at sinus arrhythmia.*)

Keep at it

If sinus arrhythmia is induced by drugs, such as morphine sulfate and other sedatives, the doctor may decide to continue to give the patient those medications. If sinus arrhythmia develops suddenly in a patient taking digoxin, notify the doctor immediately. The patient may be experiencing digoxin toxicity.

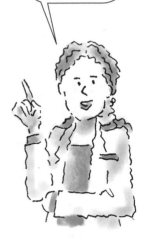

Notify the doctor if sinus arrhythmia develops suddenly in a patient taking digoxin.

Sinus bradycardia

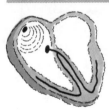

Sinus bradycardia is characterized by a sinus rate below 60 beats/ minute and a regular rhythm. It may occur normally during sleep or in a person with a well-conditioned heart — an athlete, for instance. Many athletes develop it because their well-conditioned hearts can maintain a normal stroke volume with less-than-normal effort. Sinus bradycardia also occurs normally during sleep as a result of circadian variations in heart rate.

How it happens

Sinus bradycardia usually occurs as the normal response to a reduced demand for blood flow. In this case, vagal stimulation increases and sympathetic stimulation decreases. (See *Causes of sinus bradycardia.*) As a result, automaticity (the tendency of cells to initiate their own impulses) in the SA node diminishes.

A tolerable condition?

Sinus bradycardia commonly occurs after an inferior wall MI that involves the right coronary artery, which supplies blood to the SA node. It can also result from numerous other conditions and the use of certain drugs.

The clinical significance of sinus bradycardia depends on how low the rate is and whether the patient is symptomatic. For instance, most adults can tolerate a sinus bradycardia of 45 to 59 beats/minute but are less tolerant of a rate below 45 beats/minute.

No symptoms? No problem.

Usually, sinus bradycardia is asymptomatic and insignificant. Unless the patient shows symptoms of decreased cardiac output, no treatment is necessary. (See *Treating symptomatic bradycardia,* pages 68 and 69.)

Symptoms? Problem!

When sinus bradycardia is symptomatic, however, prompt attention is critical. The heart of a patient with underlying cardiac disease may not be able to compensate for a drop in rate by increasing its stroke volume. The resulting drop in cardiac output produces such signs and symptoms as hypotension and dizziness. Bradycardia may also predispose some patients to more serious arrhythmias, such as ventricular tachycardia and ventricular fibrillation.

In a patient with acute inferior wall MI, sinus bradycardia is considered a favorable prognostic sign, unless it's accompanied by hypotension. Because sinus bradycardia rarely affects children, it's considered a poor prognostic sign in ill children.

What to look for

In sinus bradycardia, the atrial and ventricular rhythms are regular, as are their rates, except that they're both under 60 beats/minute. (See *Recognizing sinus bradycardia,* page 70.) Everything else is

(Text continues on page 70.)

Causes of sinus bradycardia

Sinus bradycardia may be caused by:
• noncardiac disorders, such as hyperkalemia, increased intracranial pressure, hypothyroidism, hypothermia, sleep, and glaucoma
• conditions producing excess vagal stimulation or decreased sympathetic stimulation, such as sleep, deep relaxation, Valsalva's maneuver, carotid sinus massage, and vomiting
• cardiac diseases, such as sinoatrial node disease, cardiomyopathy, myocarditis, myocardial ischemia, and heart block; sinus bradycardia can also occur immediately following an inferior wall myocardial infarction
• certain drugs, especially beta-adrenergic blockers, digoxin, calcium channel blockers, lithium, and antiarrhythmics, such as sotalol, amiodarone, propafenone, and quinidine.

Treating symptomatic bradycardia

The following algorithm shows the steps for treating bradycardia in a patient not in cardiac arrest.

Perform initial assessment and early interventions:
• Assess airway, breathing, and circulation.
• Secure the patient's airway noninvasively.
• Ensure that a monitor defibrillator is available.
• Assess whether invasive airway management is needed.
• Administer oxygen.
• Start an I.V. line, attach a monitor, and give I.V. fluids.
• Assess vital signs, and apply a pulse oximeter and an automatic sphygmomanometer.
• Obtain and review a 12-lead ECG.
• Obtain and review a portable chest X-ray.
• Review the patient's history.
• Perform a physical examination.
• Develop a differential diagnosis.

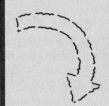

If assessment indicates bradycardia, monitor for serious signs, symptoms, and complications, including chest pain, shortness of breath, decreased level of consciousness, low blood pressure, shock, pulmonary congestion, heart failure, and acute myocardial infarction.

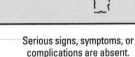

Serious signs, symptoms, or complications are absent.

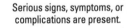

Serious signs, symptoms, or complications are present.

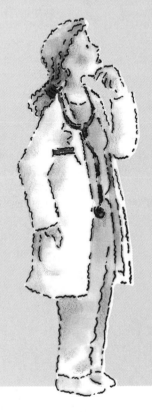

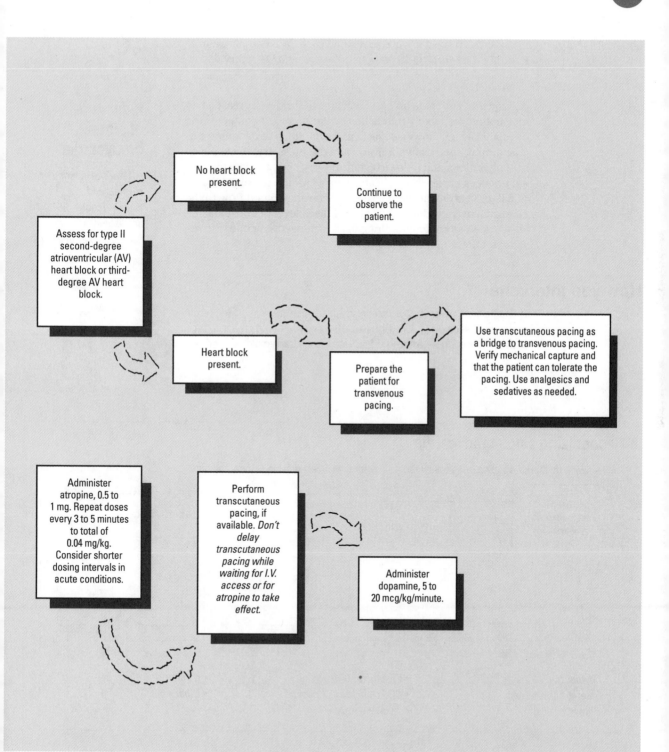

Assess for type II second-degree atrioventricular (AV) heart block or third-degree AV heart block.

No heart block present.

Continue to observe the patient.

Heart block present.

Prepare the patient for transvenous pacing.

Use transcutaneous pacing as a bridge to transvenous pacing. Verify mechanical capture and that the patient can tolerate the pacing. Use analgesics and sedatives as needed.

Administer atropine, 0.5 to 1 mg. Repeat doses every 3 to 5 minutes to total of 0.04 mg/kg. Consider shorter dosing intervals in acute conditions.

Perform transcutaneous pacing, if available. *Don't delay transcutaneous pacing while waiting for I.V. access or for atropine to take effect.*

Administer dopamine, 5 to 20 mcg/kg/minute.

normal. You'll see a P wave preceding each QRS complex and a normal PR interval, QRS complex, T wave, and QT interval.

When cardiac output gets low

As long as a patient is able to compensate for the decreased cardiac output, he's likely to remain asymptomatic. If compensatory mechanisms fail, however, signs and symptoms of declining cardiac output, such as hypotension and dizziness, usually appear.

Palpitations and pulse irregularities may occur if the patient experiences more ectopic beats, such as premature atrial, junctional, or ventricular contractions. Diminished blood flow to the cerebrum may produce signs of decreased level of consciousness (LOC) such as confusion. Bradycardia-induced syncope (Stokes-Adams attack) may also occur.

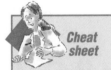

Cheat sheet

Indicators of sinus bradycardia

• *Atrial and ventricular rhythms and rates*—regular; under 60 beats/minute
• *All other parameters*—normal

How you intervene

If the patient is asymptomatic and his vital signs are stable, treatment isn't necessary. Continue to observe his heart rhythm, monitoring the progression and duration of the bradycardia. Evaluate

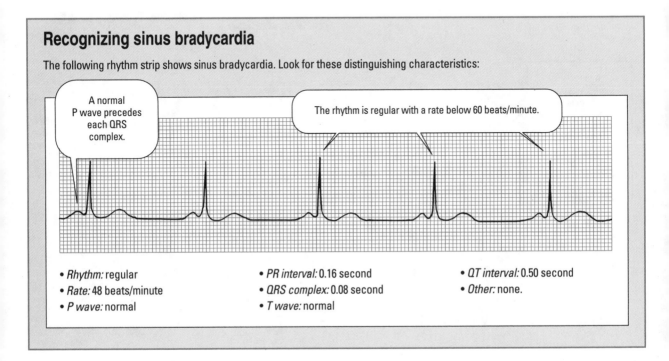

Recognizing sinus bradycardia

The following rhythm strip shows sinus bradycardia. Look for these distinguishing characteristics:

A normal P wave precedes each QRS complex.

The rhythm is regular with a rate below 60 beats/minute.

• *Rhythm:* regular
• *Rate:* 48 beats/minute
• *P wave:* normal
• *PR interval:* 0.16 second
• *QRS complex:* 0.08 second
• *T wave:* normal
• *QT interval:* 0.50 second
• *Other:* none.

his tolerance of the rhythm at rest and with activity. Review the drugs he's taking. Check with the doctor about stopping any medications that may be depressing the SA node, such as digoxin, beta-adrenergic blockers, or calcium channel blockers. Before giving those drugs, make sure the heart rate is within a safe range.

Identify and correct

If the patient is symptomatic, treatment aims to identify and correct the underlying cause. Meanwhile, the heart rate must be maintained with such drugs as atropine, epinephrine, and dopamine or with a temporary or permanent pacemaker.

Atropine is given as a 0.5- to 1-mg dose by rapid injection. The dose may be repeated every 3 to 5 minutes up to a maximum of 0.04 mg/kg total. If atropine proves ineffective, administer an epinephrine infusion at a rate of 2 to 10 mcg/minute. If low blood pressure accompanies bradycardia, administer a dopamine infusion at 5 to 20 mcg/kg/minute. Treatment of chronic, symptomatic sinus bradycardia requires insertion of a permanent pacemaker.

Check the ABCs

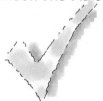

If the patient abruptly develops a significant sinus bradycardia, assess his airway, breathing, and circulation (ABCs). If these are adequate, determine whether the patient has an effective cardiac output. If not, he'll become symptomatic. (See *Clues to symptomatic bradycardia.*)

When administering atropine, be sure to give the correct dose: Doses lower than 0.5 mg can have a paradoxical effect, slowing the heart rate even further. Keep in mind that a patient with a transplanted heart won't respond to atropine and may require pacing for emergency treatment.

Clues to symptomatic bradycardia

If a patient can't tolerate bradycardia, he may develop these signs and symptoms:
- hypotension
- cool, clammy skin
- altered mental status
- dizziness
- blurred vision
- crackles, dyspnea, and an S_3 heart sound, which indicate heart failure
- chest pain
- syncope.

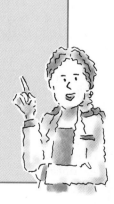

Sinus tachycardia

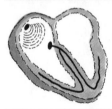

If sinus bradycardia is the tortoise of the sinus arrhythmias, sinus tachycardia is the hare. Sinus tachycardia in an adult is characterized by a sinus rate of more than 100 beats/minute. The rate rarely exceeds 180 except during strenuous exercise; the maximum rate achievable with exercise decreases with age.

How it happens

The clinical significance of sinus tachycardia depends on the underlying cause. (See *Causes of sinus tachycardia.*) The arrhythmia may be the body's response to exercise or high emotional states and may be of no clinical significance. It may also occur with hypovolemia, hemorrhage, or pain. When the stimulus for the tachycardia is removed, the arrhythmia spontaneously resolves.

Hard on the heart

Sinus tachycardia can also be a significant arrhythmia with dire consequences. Because myocardial demands for oxygen are increased at higher heart rates, tachycardia can bring on an episode of chest pain in patients with coronary artery disease.

An increase in heart rate can also be detrimental for patients with obstructive types of heart conditions, such as aortic stenosis and hypertrophic cardiomyopathy.

Sinus tachycardia occurs in about 30% of patients after acute MI and is considered a poor prognostic sign because it may be associated with massive heart damage. Persistent tachycardia may also signal impending heart failure or cardiogenic shock.

What to look for

In sinus tachycardia, atrial and ventricular rhythms are regular. (See *Recognizing sinus tachycardia.*) Both rates are equal, generally 100 to 160 beats/minute. As in sinus bradycardia, the P wave is of normal size and shape and precedes each QRS, but it may increase in amplitude. As the heart rate increases, the P wave may be superimposed on the preceding T wave and difficult to identify.

The PR interval, QRS complex, and T wave are normal. The QT interval normally shortens with tachycardia.

Pulse check!

When assessing a patient with sinus tachycardia, look for a peripheral pulse rate of more than 100 beats/minute but

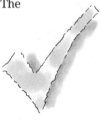

Causes of sinus tachycardia

Sinus tachycardia may be a normal response to exercise, pain, stress, fever, or strong emotions, such as fear and anxiety. It can also occur:

• in certain cardiac conditions, such as heart failure, cardiogenic shock, and pericarditis
• as a compensatory mechanism in shock, anemia, respiratory distress, pulmonary embolism, sepsis, and hyperthyroidism
• when taking such drugs as atropine, isoproterenol, aminophylline, dopamine, dobutamine, epinephrine, alcohol, caffeine, nicotine, and amphetamines.

with a regular rhythm. Usually, the patient will be asymptomatic. However, if his cardiac output falls and compensatory mechanisms fail, he may experience hypotension, syncope, and blurred vision. (See *What happens in tachycardia*, page 74.)

He may report chest pain and palpitations, commonly described as a pounding chest or a sensation of skipped heartbeats. He may also report a sense of nervousness or anxiety. If heart failure develops, he may exhibit crackles, an extra heart sound (S_3), and jugular vein distention.

How you intervene

No treatment of sinus tachycardia is necessary if the patient is asymptomatic or if the rhythm is the result of physical exertion. In other cases, the underlying cause of the arrhythmia may be treated. For example, if the tachycardia is caused by hemorrhage, treatment includes stopping the bleeding and replacing blood and fluid.

Slow it down

If tachycardia leads to cardiac ischemia, treatment may include medications to slow the heart rate. The most commonly used drugs include beta-adrenergic blockers, such as metoprolol

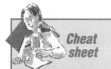

Cheat sheet

Indicators of sinus tachycardia

• *Atrial and ventricular rhythms and rates*— regular; both equal, generally 100 to 160 beats/minute
• *PR interval*—normal
• *QRS complex*—normal
• *T wave*—normal
• *QT interval*—shortened

Recognizing sinus tachycardia

The following rhythm strip illustrates sinus tachycardia. Look for these distinguishing characteristics:

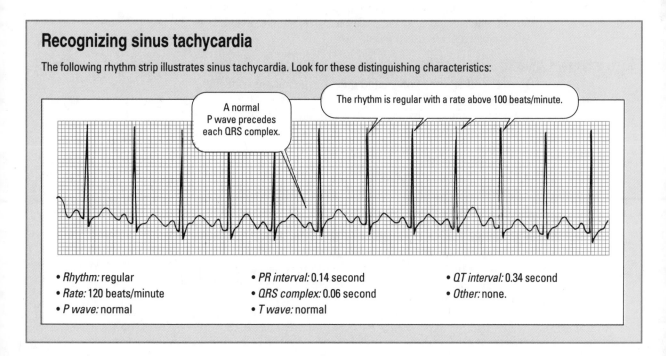

A normal P wave precedes each QRS complex.

The rhythm is regular with a rate above 100 beats/minute.

• *Rhythm:* regular
• *Rate:* 120 beats/minute
• *P wave:* normal
• *PR interval:* 0.14 second
• *QRS complex:* 0.06 second
• *T wave:* normal
• *QT interval:* 0.34 second
• *Other:* none.

What happens in tachycardia

Tachycardia can lower cardiac output by reducing ventricular filling time and the amount of blood pumped by the ventricles during each contraction. Normally, ventricular volume reaches 120 to 130 ml during diastole. In tachycardia, decreased ventricular volume leads to hypotension and decreased peripheral perfusion.

As cardiac output plummets, arterial pressure and peripheral perfusion decrease. Tachycardia worsens myocardial ischemia by increasing the heart's demand for oxygen and reducing the duration of diastole — the period of greatest coronary flow.

(Lopressor) and atenolol (Tenormin), and calcium channel blockers such as verapamil (Isoptin).

The goal of an intervention for the patient with sinus tachycardia is to maintain adequate cardiac output and tissue perfusion and to identify and correct the underlying cause.

Getting at the history

Check the patient's medication history. Over-the-counter sympathomimetic agents, which mimic the effects of the sympathetic nervous system, may contribute to the sinus tachycardia. These agents may be contained in nose drops and cold formulas.

You should also ask about the patient's use of caffeine, nicotine, alcohol, and such illicit drugs as cocaine and amphetamines, any of which can trigger tachycardia. Advise him to avoid these substances if he has used them.

More steps to take

Here are other steps you should take for the patient with sinus tachycardia.

• Because sinus tachycardia can lead to injury of the heart muscle, check for chest pain or angina. Also assess for signs and symptoms of heart failure, including crackles, an S_3 heart sound, and jugular vein distention.

• Monitor intake and output as well as daily weight.

• Check the patient's LOC to assess cerebral perfusion.

• Provide the patient with a calm environment. Help to reduce fear and anxiety, which can fuel the arrhythmia.

• Teach about procedures and treatments. Include relaxation techniques in the information you provide.

• Be aware that a sudden onset of sinus tachycardia after an MI may signal extension of the infarction. Prompt recognition is vital so treatment can be started.

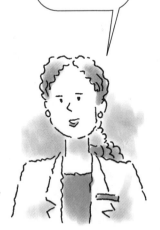

Advise the patient to avoid caffeine, nicotine, alcohol, and illicit drugs.

Sinus arrest

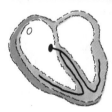

A disorder of impulse formation, sinus arrest is caused by a lack of electrical activity in the atrium, a condition called atrial standstill. (See *Causes of sinus arrest.*) During atrial standstill, the atria aren't stimulated and an entire PQRST complex will be missing from the ECG strip.

Except for this missing complex, or pause, the ECG usually remains normal. Atrial standstill is called sinus pause when one or two beats aren't formed and sinus arrest when three or more beats aren't formed.

Sinus arrest closely resembles third-degree SA block, also called exit block, on the ECG strip. (See *Understanding sinoatrial blocks,* pages 76 and 77.)

How it happens

Sinus arrest occurs when the SA node fails to generate an impulse. Such failure may result from a number of conditions, including acute infection, heart disease, and vagal stimulation. Sinus arrest may be associated with sick sinus syndrome.

The clinical significance of sinus arrest depends on the patient's symptoms. If the pauses are short and infrequent, the patient will most likely be asymptomatic and won't require treatment. He may have a normal sinus rhythm for days or weeks between episodes of sinus arrest. He may not be able to feel the arrhythmias at all.

Pauses of 2 to 3 seconds normally occur in healthy adults during sleep and occasionally in patients with increased vagal tone or hypersensitive carotid sinus disease.

Too many for too long

If sinus arrest is frequent and prolonged, however, the patient will most likely have symptoms. The arrhythmias can produce syncope or near-syncopal episodes usually within 7 seconds of asystole.

During a prolonged pause, the patient may fall and injure himself. Other situations may be just as serious. For instance, a symptomatic arrhythmia that occurs while the patient is driving a car could result in a fatal accident.

Causes of sinus arrest

The following conditions can cause sinus arrest:
• sinus node disease, such as fibrosis and idiopathic degeneration
• increased vagal tone, as occurs with Valsalva's maneuver, carotid sinus massage, and vomiting
• digoxin, quinidine, procainamide and salicylates, especially if given at toxic levels
• excessive doses of beta-adrenergic blockers, such as metoprolol and propranolol
• cardiac disorders, such as chronic coronary artery disease, acute myocarditis, cardiomyopathy, and hypertensive heart disease
• acute inferior wall myocardial infarction.

Understanding sinoatrial blocks

In sinoatrial (SA) block, the SA node discharges impulses at regular intervals. Some of those impulses, though, are delayed on their way to the atria. Based on the length of the delay, SA blocks are divided into three categories: first-, second-, and third-degree. Second-degree block is further divided into type I (Wenckebach) and type II.

First-degree SA block consists of a delay between the firing of the sinus node and depolarization of the atria. Because the ECG doesn't show sinus node activity, you can't detect first-degree SA block. However, you can detect the other three types of SA block.

Second-degree type I block

In second-degree type I block, conduction time between the sinus node and the surrounding atrial tissue becomes progressively longer until an entire cycle is dropped. The pause is less than twice the shortest P-P interval.

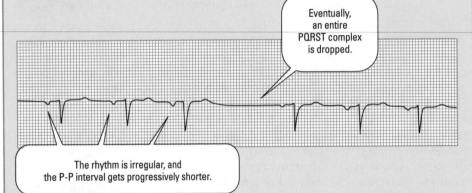

Eventually, an entire PQRST complex is dropped.

The rhythm is irregular, and the P-P interval gets progressively shorter.

Second-degree type II block

In second-degree type II block, conduction time between the sinus node and atrial tissue is normal until an impulse is blocked. The duration of the pause is a multiple of the P-P interval.

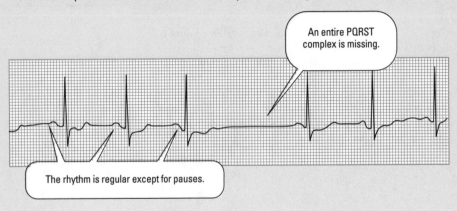

An entire PQRST complex is missing.

The rhythm is regular except for pauses.

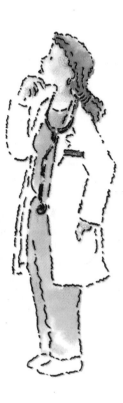

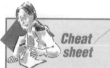

Understanding sinoatrial blocks (continued)

Third-degree block

In third-degree block, some impulses are blocked, causing long sinus pauses. The pause isn't a multiple of the sinus rhythm. On an ECG, third-degree SA block looks similar to sinus arrest but results from a different cause.

Third-degree SA block is caused by a failure to conduct impulses; sinus arrest results from failure to form impulses. Failure in each case causes atrial activity to stop.

In sinus arrest, the pause commonly ends with a junctional escape beat. In third-degree block, the pause lasts for an indefinite period and ends with a sinus beat.

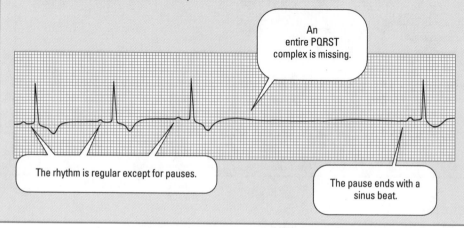

An entire PQRST complex is missing.

The rhythm is regular except for pauses.

The pause ends with a sinus beat.

Indicators of sinus arrest

• *Atrial and ventricular rhythms*—regular, except for missing complex
• *Atrial and ventricular rates*—equal and usually within normal limits; may vary as a result of pauses
• *P wave*—normal and constant when P wave is present; not measurable when P wave is absent
• *QRS complex*—normal when present; absent during pause
• *T wave*—normal when present; absent during pause
• *QT interval*—normal when present; absent during pause

What to look for

When assessing for sinus pause, you'll find that atrial and ventricular rhythms are regular except for a missing complex at the onset of atrial standstill. (See *Recognizing sinus arrest*, page 78.) The atrial and ventricular rates are equal and usually within normal limits. The rate may vary, however, as a result of the pauses.

Of normal size and shape, a P wave precedes each QRS complex but is absent during a pause. The PR interval is normal and constant when the P wave is present and not measurable when absent. The QRS complex, the T wave, and the QT interval are normal when present and are absent during a pause.

You might see junctional escape beats, including premature atrial, junctional, or ventricular contractions. With sinus arrest, the length of the pause is not a multiple of the previous R-R intervals.

Recognizing sinus arrest

The following rhythm strip illustrates sinus arrest. Look for these distinguishing characteristics:

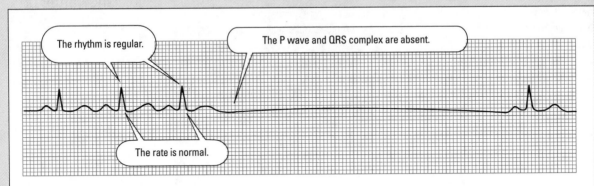

The rhythm is regular.

The P wave and QRS complex are absent.

The rate is normal.

- *Rhythm:* regular, except for the missing PQRST complexes
- *Rate:* 40 beats/minute
- *P wave:* normal; missing during pause

- *PR interval:* 0.20 second
- *QRS complex:* 0.08 second, absent during pause
- *T wave:* normal, absent during pause

- *QT interval:* 0.40 second, absent during pause
- *Other:* none.

The pause that decreases

You won't be able to detect a pulse or heart sounds when sinus arrest occurs. Usually, the patient will be asymptomatic. Recurrent pauses may cause signs of decreased cardiac output, such as low blood pressure, altered mental status, and cool, clammy skin. The patient may also complain of dizziness or blurred vision.

How you intervene

An asymptomatic patient needs no treatment. For a patient displaying mild symptoms, treatment focuses on maintaining cardiac output and identifying the cause of the sinus arrest. That may involve stopping medications that contribute to SA node suppression, such as digoxin, beta-adrenergic blockers, and calcium channel blockers.

Atropine

A patient who develops signs of circulatory collapse needs immediate treatment. As with sinus bradycardia, emergency treatment includes administration of

STAT!

Syncope and sinus arrest

A patient with sinus arrest is at risk for syncope. Ask your patient whether he has ever passed out or felt as if he were going to pass out.

Also ask about a history of falls. If he has passed out or if he has a history of falls, obtain a detailed description of each episode, including where and how the syncope occurred.

Asking questions

If possible, check with friends and family members who witnessed the episodes to find out what happened and how long the patient remained unconscious each time.

The information you gather may help determine whether a vagal mechanism was involved. The presence of syncope or sinus pauses on an electrocardiogram may indicate the need for further electrophysiologic evaluation.

atropine or epinephrine and insertion of a temporary pacemaker. A permanent pacemaker may be implanted for long-term management.

The goal for the patient with sinus arrest is to maintain adequate cardiac output and perfusion. Be sure to record and document the frequency and duration of pauses. Determine whether a pause is the result of sinus arrest or SA block.

Don't let sleeping pauses lie

Examine the circumstances under which sinus pauses occur. A sinus pause may be insignificant if detected while the patient is sleeping. If the pauses are recurrent, assess the patient for evidence of decreased cardiac output, such as altered mental status, low blood pressure, and cool, clammy skin.

Ask him whether he's dizzy or light-headed or has blurred vision. Does he feel as if he has passed out? If so, he may be experiencing syncope from a prolonged sinus arrest. (See *Syncope and sinus arrest.*)

Document the patient's vital signs and how he feels during pauses as well as what activities he was involved in when they occurred. Activities that increase vagal stimulation, such as Valsalva's maneuver or vomiting, increase the likelihood of sinus pauses.

When matters get even worse

Assess for a progression of the arrhythmia. Notify the doctor immediately if the patient becomes unstable. Lower the head of the bed and administer atropine or epinephrine, as ordered or as your facility's policy directs. Withhold medications that may contribute to sinus pauses and check with the doctor about whether those drugs should be continued.

If appropriate, be alert for signs of digoxin, quinidine, or procainamide toxicity. Obtain a serum digoxin level and a serum electrolyte level. If a pacemaker is implanted, give the patient discharge instructions about pacemaker care.

Sick sinus syndrome

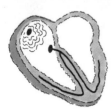

Also called sinus nodal dysfunction, sick sinus syndrome refers to a wide spectrum of SA node abnormalities. The syndrome is caused by disturbances in the way impulses are generated or the inability to conduct impulses to the atrium.

Sick sinus syndrome usually shows up as bradycardia, with episodes of sinus arrest and SA block interspersed with sudden, brief periods of rapid atrial fibrillation. Patients are also prone to paroxysms of other atrial tachyarrhythmias, such as atrial flutter and ectopic atrial tachycardia, a condition sometimes referred to as bradycardia-tachycardia (or brady-tachy) syndrome.

Most patients with sick sinus syndrome are older than age 60, but anyone can develop the arrhythmia. It's rare in children except after open-heart surgery that results in SA node damage. The arrhythmia affects men and women equally. The onset is progressive, insidious, and chronic.

How it happens

Sick sinus syndrome results either from a dysfunction of the sinus node's automaticity or from abnormal conduction or blockages of impulses coming out of the nodal region. (See *Causes of sick sinus syndrome.*) These conditions, in turn, stem from a degeneration of the area's autonomic nervous system and partial destruction of the sinus node, as may occur with an interrupted blood supply after an inferior wall MI.

Blocked exits

In addition, certain conditions can affect the atrial wall surrounding the SA node and cause exit blocks. Conditions that cause inflammation or degeneration of atrial tissue can also lead to sick sinus syndrome. In many patients, though, the exact cause of sick sinus syndrome is never identified.

Prognosis of the diagnosis

The significance of sick sinus syndrome depends on the patient's age, the presence of other diseases, and the type and duration of the specific arrhythmias that occur. If atrial fibrillation is involved,

Causes of sick sinus syndrome

Sick sinus syndrome may result from:
• conditions leading to fibrosis of the sinoatrial (SA) node, such as increased age, atherosclerotic heart disease, hypertension, and cardiomyopathy
• trauma to the SA node caused by open heart surgery (especially valvular surgery), pericarditis, or rheumatic heart disease
• autonomic disturbances affecting autonomic innervation, such as hypervagatonia or degeneration of the autonomic system
• cardioactive medications, such as digoxin, beta-adrenergic blockers, and calcium channel blockers.

the prognosis is worse, most likely because of the risk of thromboembolic complications.

If prolonged pauses are involved with sick sinus syndrome, syncope may occur. The length of a pause significant enough to cause syncope varies with the patient's age, posture at the time, and cerebrovascular status. Consider significant any pause that lasts at least 2 to 3 seconds.

Long-term problems

A significant part of the diagnosis is whether the patient experiences symptoms while the disturbance occurs. Because the syndrome is progressive and chronic, a symptomatic patient will need lifelong treatment. In addition, thromboembolism may develop as a complication of sick sinus syndrome, possibly resulting in stroke or peripheral embolization.

What to look for

Sick sinus syndrome encompasses several potential rhythm disturbances that may be intermittent or chronic. (See *Recognizing sick sinus syndrome*, page 82.) Those rhythm disturbances include one or a combination of the following:
- sinus bradycardia
- SA block
- sinus arrest
- sinus bradycardia alternating with sinus tachycardia
- episodes of atrial tachyarrhythmias, such as atrial fibrillation and atrial flutter
- failure of the sinus node to increase heart rate with exercise.

Check for speed bumps

Also look for an irregular rhythm with sinus pauses and abrupt rate changes. Atrial and ventricular rates may be fast, slow, or alternating periods of fast rates and slow rates interrupted by pauses.

The P wave varies with the rhythm and usually precedes each QRS complex. The PR interval is usually within normal limits but varies with changes in the rhythm. The QRS complex and T wave are usually normal, as is the QT interval, which may vary with rhythm changes.

No set pattern

The patient's pulse rate may be fast, slow, or normal, and the rhythm may be regular or irregular. You can usually detect an irregularity on the monitor or when palpating the pulse, which may feel inappropriately slow, then rapid.

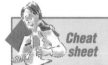

Cheat sheet

Indicators of sick sinus syndrome

- *Rhythm*—irregular with sinus pauses and abrupt rate changes
- *Atrial and ventricular rates*—may be fast, slow, or combination of both
- *P wave*—varies with rhythm and usually precedes QRS complex
- *PR interval*—usually within normal limits; varies with changes in rhythm
- *QRS complex*— normal
- *T wave*—normal
- *QT interval*—normal; may vary with rhythm changes

Recognizing sick sinus syndrome

This rhythm strip illustrates sick sinus syndrome. Look for these distinguishing characteristics:

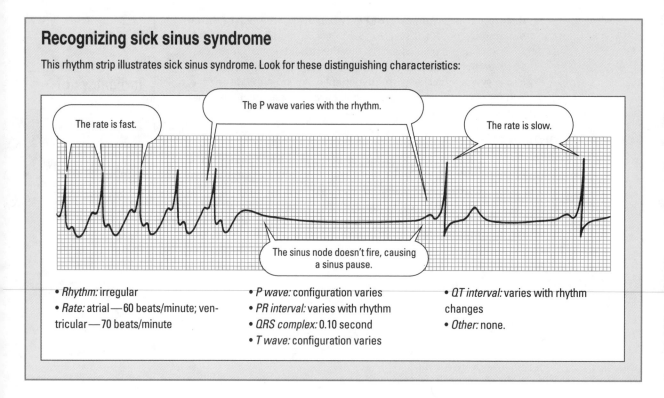

The rate is fast.

The P wave varies with the rhythm.

The rate is slow.

The sinus node doesn't fire, causing a sinus pause.

- *Rhythm:* irregular
- *Rate:* atrial—60 beats/minute; ventricular—70 beats/minute

- *P wave:* configuration varies
- *PR interval:* varies with rhythm
- *QRS complex:* 0.10 second
- *T wave:* configuration varies

- *QT interval:* varies with rhythm changes
- *Other:* none.

If you monitor the patient's heart rate during exercise or exertion, you may observe an inappropriate response to exercise such as a failure of the heart rate to increase. You may also detect episodes of brady-tachy syndrome, atrial flutter, atrial fibrillation, SA block, or sinus arrest on the monitor.

Extra sounds

Other assessment findings depend on the patient's condition. For instance, he may have crackles in the lungs, an S₃ heart sound, or a dilated and displaced left ventricular apical impulse if he has underlying cardiomyopathy.

The patient may show signs and symptoms of decreased cardiac output, such as hypotension, blurred vision, and syncope, a common experience with this arrhythmia.

How you intervene

As with other sinus node arrhythmias, no treatment is necessary if the patient is asymptomatic. If the patient is symptomatic, howev-

Recognizing an embolism

When caring for a patient with sick sinus syndrome, be alert for signs and symptoms of an embolism, especially if the patient has atrial fibrillation. Any clots that form in the heart can break off and travel through the bloodstream, blocking the blood supply to the lungs, heart, brain, kidneys, intestines, or other organs.

Assess early

Assess the patient for neurologic changes, such as confusion, visual disturbances, weakness, chest pain, dyspnea, tachypnea, tachycardia, and acute onset of pain. Early recognition allows for prompt treatment.

er, treatment aims to alleviate signs and symptoms and correct the underlying cause of the arrhythmia.

Atropine or epinephrine may be given initially for an acute attack. A pacemaker may be used until the underlying disorder resolves. Tachyarrhythmias may be treated with antiarrhythmic medications, such as metoprolol and digoxin.

Drugs don't always help

Unfortunately, medications used to suppress tachyarrhythmias may worsen underlying SA node disease and bradyarrhythmias. The patient may need anticoagulants if he develops sudden bursts, or paroxysms, of atrial fibrillation. The anticoagulants help prevent thromboembolism and stroke, a complication of the condition. (See *Recognizing an embolism.*)

Watch and document

When caring for a patient with sick sinus syndrome, monitor and document all arrhythmias he experiences and signs or symptoms he develops. Assess how his rhythm responds to activity and pain and look for changes in the rhythm.

Watch the patient carefully after starting calcium channel blockers, beta-adrenergic blockers, or other antiarrhythmic medications. If treatment includes anticoagulant therapy and the insertion of a pacemaker, make sure the patient and his family receive appropriate instruction.

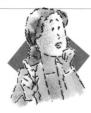

Quick quiz

1. A patient with symptomatic sinus bradycardia at a rate of 40 beats/minute typically experiences:
   A.   high blood pressure.
   B.   chest pain and dyspnea.
   C.   facial flushing and ataxia.

Answer: B. A patient with symptomatic bradycardia suffers from low cardiac output, which may produce chest pain and dyspnea. The patient may also have crackles, an S_3 heart sound, and a sudden onset of confusion.

2. For a patient with symptomatic sinus bradycardia, appropriate nursing interventions include establishing I.V. access to administer:
   A.   atropine.
   B.   anticoagulants.
   C.   a calcium channel blocker.

Answer: A. Atropine or epinephrine are standard treatments for sinus bradycardia.

3. A monitor shows an irregular rhythm and a rate that increases and decreases in consistent cycles. This rhythm most likely represents:
   A.   sinus arrest.
   B.   sinus bradycardia.
   C.   sinus arrhythmia.

Answer: C. In sinus arrhythmia, common among young people, the heart rate varies with the respiratory cycle and is rarely treated.

4. Treatment for symptomatic sick sinus syndrome includes:
   A.   beta-adrenergic blockers.
   B.   ventilatory support.
   C.   pacemaker insertion.

Answer: C. A pacemaker is commonly used to maintain a steady heart rate in patients with sick sinus syndrome.

5. Persistent tachycardia in a patient who has had an MI may signal:
   A.   chronic sick sinus syndrome.
   B.   pulmonary embolism or stroke.
   C.   impending heart failure or cardiogenic shock.

Answer: C. Sinus tachycardia occurs in about 30% of patients after acute MI and is considered a poor prognostic sign because it may be associated with massive heart damage.

6. Beta-adrenergic blockers, such as metoprolol and atenolol, and calcium channel blockers such as verapamil may be used to treat the sinus node arrhythmia:
   A. sinus bradycardia.
   B. sinus tachycardia.
   C. sinus arrest.

Answer: B. Beta-adrenergic blockers and calcium channel blockers may be used to treat sinus tachycardia.

Test strips

Try these test strips. Answer the questions accompanying each strip; then check your answers with ours.

7. In the rhythm strip below, the rhythm is regular except during a pause; the atrial and ventricular rates are 50 beats/minute; the P wave is of normal size and configuration, except when missing during a pause; the PR interval is 0.16 second; the QRS complex is 0.10 second and is of normal size and configuration, except when missing during a pause; the T wave is normal except when missing during a pause; the QT interval is 0.42 second; and the pause isn't a multiple of a previous sinus rhythm. You would interpret the strip as:
   A. sinus bradycardia.
   B. sinus arrest, or third-degree SA block.
   C. sick sinus syndrome.

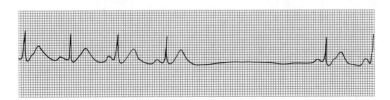

Answer: B. The strip shows sinus arrest, or third-degree SA block.

8. In the rhythm strip below, the atrial and ventricular rhythms are regular at 110 beats/minute, the P wave is normal, the PR interval is 0.14 second, the QRS complex is 0.08 second and of normal size and configuration, the T wave is normal, and the QT interval is 0.36 second. You would interpret the strip as:

A. sinus tachycardia.
B. sinus arrhythmia.
C. sick sinus syndrome.

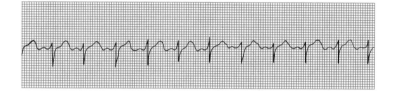

Answer: A. The strip shows sinus tachycardia.

9. Your patient's monitor produces the rhythm strip shown below. After examining its characteristics, you identify the rhythm as:

A. normal sinus rhythm.
B. sinus arrhythmia.
C. sick sinus syndrome.

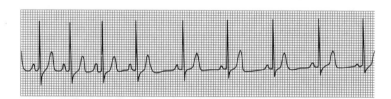

Answer: B. The strip shows sinus arrhythmia. The atrial and ventricular rhythms are irregular with rates of 90 beats/minute; the P wave is normal; the PR interval is 0.12 second; the QRS complex is 0.10 second and normal; the T wave is normal; and the QT interval is 0.30 second.

Scoring

☆☆☆ If you answered all nine questions correctly, WOW! You deserve to head down to the nearest club and tachy-brady the night away!

☆☆ If you answered six to eight questions correctly, super! When you get to the club, you can lead the dance parade!

☆ If you answered fewer than six questions correctly, great. A few lessons and you'll be tachy-brading with the best of 'em!

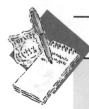

⑤

Atrial arrhythmias

Just the facts

This chapter will show you how to identify and care for patients with atrial arrhythmias, including premature atrial contractions, atrial tachycardia, atrial flutter, and atrial fibrillation. In this chapter, you'll learn:

♦ causes of atrial arrhythmias

♦ signs and symptoms of atrial arrhythmias

♦ effects atrial arrhythmias have on a patient

♦ nursing interventions and medical treatments appropriate for atrial arrhythmias.

A look at atrial arrhythmias

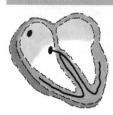

Atrial arrhythmias, the most common cardiac rhythm disturbances, result from impulses originating in areas outside the sinoatrial (SA) node. These arrhythmias can affect ventricular filling time and diminish the strength of the atrial kick, a contraction that normally provides the ventricles with about 30% of their blood.

Triple play

Atrial arrhythmias are thought to result from three mechanisms—altered automaticity, circus reentry, and afterdepolarization. Let's take a look at each cause and review specific atrial arrhythmias:
• *Altered automaticity*— An increase in the automaticity (the ability of cardiac cells to initiate impulses on their own) of the atrial fibers can trigger abnormal impulses. Causes of increased automaticity include extracellular factors, such as hypoxia, hypocalcemia, and digoxin toxicity, and conditions in which the function of the heart's normal pacemaker, the SA node, is dimin-

ished. For example, increased vagal tone or hypokalemia can increase the refractory period of the SA node and allow atrial fibers to fire impulses.

• *Reentry*—In reentry, an impulse is delayed along a slow conduction pathway. Despite the delay, the impulse remains active enough to produce another impulse during myocardial repolarization. Reentry may occur with coronary artery disease cardiomyopathy or myocardial infarction (MI).

• *Afterdepolarization*—Afterdepolarization can occur with cell injury, digoxin toxicity, and other conditions. An injured cell sometimes only partly repolarizes. Partial repolarization can lead to a repetitive ectopic firing called triggered activity. The depolarization produced by triggered activity is known as afterdepolarization and can lead to atrial or ventricular tachycardia. Let's examine each atrial arrhythmia in detail.

Premature atrial contraction

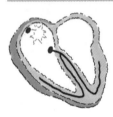

Premature atrial contractions (PACs) originate outside the SA node and usually result from an irritable spot, or focus, in the atria that takes over as pacemaker for one or more beats. The SA node fires an impulse, but then an irritable focus jumps in, firing its own impulse before the SA node can fire again.

PACs may or may not be conducted through the atrioventricular (AV) node and the rest of the heart, depending on their prematurity and the status of the AV and intraventricular conduction system. Nonconducted or blocked PACs don't trigger a QRS complex.

How it happens

PACs, which commonly occur in a normal heart, can be triggered by alcohol, cigarettes, anxiety, fatigue, fever, and infectious diseases. Patients who eliminate or control those factors can correct the arrhythmias.

PACs may also be associated with coronary or valvular heart disease, acute respiratory failure, hypoxia, pulmonary disease, digoxin toxicity, and certain electrolyte imbalances.

PACs are rarely dangerous in patients who don't have heart disease. In fact, they commonly cause no symptoms and can go unrecognized for years. The patient may perceive PACs as normal palpitations or skipped beats.

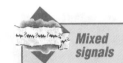

Mixed signals

Nonconducted PACs and second-degree AV block

Don't confuse nonconducted PACs with type II second-degree AV block. In type II second-degree AV block, the P-P interval is regular. A nonconducted PAC, however, is an atrial impulse that arrives early to the AV node, when the node isn't yet repolarized.

As a result, the premature P wave fails to be conducted to the ventricle. The rhythm strip below shows a P wave embedded in the preceding T wave.

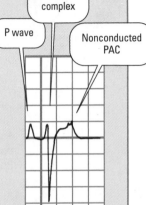

QRS complex

P wave

Nonconducted PAC

Early warning sign

However, in patients with heart disease, PACs may lead to more serious arrhythmias, such as atrial fibrillation and atrial flutter. In a patient with an acute MI, PACs can serve as an early sign of heart failure or an electrolyte imbalance. PACs can also result from the release of the neurohormone catecholamine during episodes of pain or anxiety.

What to look for

The hallmark electrocardiogram (ECG) characteristic of a PAC is a premature P wave with an abnormal configuration when compared with a sinus P wave. (See *Nonconducted PACs and second-degree AV block.*)

When the PAC is conducted, the QRS complex appears similar to the underlying QRS complex. PACs are commonly followed by a pause.

The PAC depolarizes the SA node early, causing it to reset itself and disrupt the normal cycle. The next sinus beat occurs sooner than it normally would, causing the P-P interval between two normal beats that have been interrupted by a PAC to be shorter than three consecutive sinus beats, an occurrence referred to as noncompensatory. (See *Recognizing premature atrial contractions*, page 90.)

Lost in the T

When examining a PAC on an ECG, look for irregular atrial and ventricular rates. The underlying rhythm may be regular. The P wave is premature and abnormally shaped and may be lost in the previous T wave, distorting that wave's configuration. (The T wave might be bigger or have an extra bump.) Varying configurations of the P wave indicate more than one ectopic site.

The PR interval is usually normal but may be shortened or slightly prolonged, depending on the origin of the ectopic focus. If no QRS complex follows the premature P wave, a nonconducted PAC has occurred.

PACs may occur in bigeminy (every other beat is a PAC), trigeminy (every third beat is a PAC), or couplets (two PACs at a time).

The patient may have an irregular peripheral or apical pulse rhythm when the PACs occur. He may complain of palpitations, skipped beats, or a fluttering sensation. In a patient with heart disease, signs and symptoms of decreased cardiac output—such as hypotension and syncope—may occur.

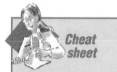

Cheat sheet

Indicators of PAC

• *Atrial and ventricular rates*—irregular
• *P wave*—premature with an abnormal configuration; may be buried in the previous T wave
• *PR interval*—usually normal; may be slightly shortened or prolonged
• *QRS complex*—similar to the underlying QRS complex when PAC is conducted
• *QRS complex*—may not follow the premature P wave when a nonconducted PAC occurs

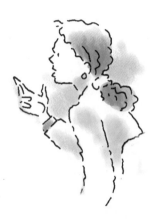

Recognizing premature atrial contractions

The following rhythm strip illustrates premature atrial contractions (PACs). Look for these distinguishing characteristics:

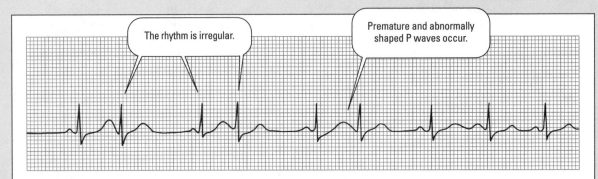

The rhythm is irregular.

Premature and abnormally shaped P waves occur.

- *Rhythm:* irregular
- *Rate:* 90 beats/minute
- *P wave:* abnormal with PAC; some lost in previous T wave

- *PR interval:* 0.20 second
- *QRS complex:* 0.08 second
- *T wave:* abnormal with some embedded P waves

- *QT interval:* 0.32 second
- *Other:* noncompensatory pause.

How you intervene

Most patients who are asymptomatic don't need treatment. If the patient is symptomatic, however, treatment may focus on eliminating the cause, such as caffeine and alcohol. People who have frequent PACs may be treated with drugs that prolong the refractory period of the atria. Those drugs include digoxin, procainamide, and quinidine.

When caring for a patient with PACs, assess him to help determine what is triggering the ectopic beats. Tailor your patient teaching to help the patient correct or avoid the underlying cause. For example, the patient might need to avoid caffeine or smoking or learn stress reduction techniques to lessen his anxiety.

If the patient has ischemic or valvular heart disease, monitor him for signs and symptoms of heart failure, electrolyte imbalances, and the development of more severe atrial arrhythmias.

PACs may be caused by too much caffeine or alcohol.

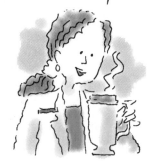

Atrial tachycardia

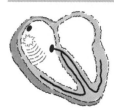

Atrial tachycardia is a supraventricular tachycardia, which means the impulses driving the rapid rhythm originate above the ventricles. Atrial tachycardia has an atrial rate from 150 to 250 beats/minute. The rapid rate shortens diastole, resulting in a loss of atrial kick, reduced cardiac output, reduced coronary perfusion, and ischemic myocardial changes.

Three types of atrial tachycardia exist: atrial tachycardia with block, multifocal atrial tachycardia (or chaotic atrial rhythm), and paroxysmal atrial tachycardia (PAT).

How it happens

Atrial tachycardia can occur in patients with normal hearts. In those cases, the condition is commonly related to excessive use of caffeine or other stimulants, marijuana use, electrolyte imbalances, hypoxia, and physical or psychological stress. However, this arrhythmia is usually associated with primary or secondary cardiac problems.

Cardiac conditions that can cause atrial tachycardia include MI, cardiomyopathy, congenital anomalies, Wolff-Parkinson-White syndrome, and valvular heart disease. This rhythm may also be a component of sick sinus syndrome. Other problems resulting in atrial tachycardia include cor pulmonale, hyperthyroidism, systemic hypertension, and digoxin toxicity, which is the most common cause of atrial tachycardia. (See *Signs of digoxin toxicity.*)

An ominous sign?

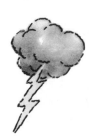

In a healthy person, atrial tachycardia is usually benign. However, this rhythm may be a forerunner of a more serious ventricular arrhythmia, especially if it occurs in a patient with an underlying heart condition.

The increased ventricular rate of atrial tachycardia results in a decrease in the time allowed for the ventricles to fill, an increase in myocardial oxygen consumption, and a decrease in oxygen supply. Angina, heart failure, ischemic myocardial changes, and even MI can occur as a result.

What to look for

Atrial tachycardia is characterized by three or more successive ectopic atrial beats at a rate of 140 to 250 beats/minute. The P wave is usually upright, if visible, and followed by a QRS complex.

Signs of digoxin toxicity

With digoxin toxicity, atrial tachycardia isn't the only change you might see in your patient. Be alert for the following signs and symptoms, especially if the patient is taking digoxin and his potassium level is low or he's also taking amiodarone. Both combinations can increase the risk of digoxin toxicity.

- *CNS:* fatigue, general muscle weakness, agitation, hallucinations
- *EENT:* yellow-green halos around visual images, blurred vision
- *GI:* anorexia, nausea, vomiting
- *CV:* arrhythmias (most commonly, conduction disturbances with or without AV block, premature ventricular contractions, and supraventricular arrhythmias), increased severity of heart failure, hypotension (Digoxin's toxic effects on the heart may be life-threatening and always require immediate attention.)

Keep in mind that atrial beats may be conducted on a 1:1 basis into the ventricles (meaning that each P wave has a QRS complex), so atrial and ventricular rates will be equal. In other cases, atrial beats may be conducted only periodically, meaning there is a block in the AV conduction system. The block keeps the ventricles from receiving every impulse.

Think of the AV node as a gatekeeper or doorman. Sometimes it lets atrial impulses through to the ventricles regularly (every other impulse, for instance), and sometimes it lets them in irregularly (two impulses might get through, for instance, and then three, and then one).

Fast but regular

When assessing a rhythm strip for atrial tachycardia, you'll see that atrial rhythm is always regular, and ventricular rhythm is regular when the block is constant and irregular when it isn't. (See *Recognizing atrial tachycardia.*) The rate consists of three or more successive ectopic atrial beats at a rate of 140 to 250 beats/minute. The ventricular rate will vary according to the AV conduction ratio.

The P wave has a 1:1 ratio with the QRS complex unless a block is present. The P wave may not be discernible because of

---

Recognizing atrial tachycardia

The following rhythm strip shows atrial tachycardia. Look for these distinguishing characteristics:

The rhythm is regular.

The P wave hides in the preceding T wave.

The rate is between 150 and 250 beats/minute.

- *Rhythm:* regular
- *Rate:* 210 beats/minute
- *P wave:* hidden in T wave
- *PR interval:* not visible
- *QRS complex:* 0.10 second
- *T wave:* inverted
- *QT interval:* 0.20 second
- *Other:* T-wave changes (inversion) indicate ischemia.

the rapid rate and may be hidden in the previous ST segment or T wave. You may not be able to measure the PR interval if the P wave can't be distinguished from the preceding T wave.

The QRS complex is usually normal, unless the impulses are being conducted abnormally through the ventricles. (See *Identifying types of atrial tachycardia*.) The T wave may be normal or inverted if ischemia is present. The QT interval is usually within normal limits but may be shorter because of the rapid rate. ST-segment and T-wave changes may appear if ischemia occurs with a prolonged arrhythmia.

Check out the outward signs

The patient with atrial tachycardia will have a rapid apical or peripheral pulse rate. The rhythm may be regular or irregular,

---

Identifying types of atrial tachycardia

Atrial tachycardia comes in three varieties. Here's a quick rundown of each.

Atrial tachycardia with block
Atrial tachycardia with block is caused by increased automaticity of the atrial tissue. As the atrial rate speeds up and atrioventricular (AV) conduction becomes impaired, a 2:1 block typically occurs. Occasionally a type I (Wenckebach) second-degree AV block may be seen.

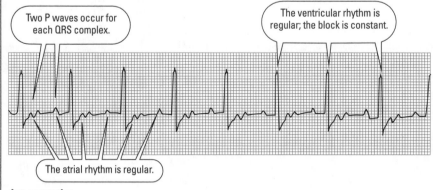

Two P waves occur for each QRS complex.

The ventricular rhythm is regular; the block is constant.

The atrial rhythm is regular.

Interpretation
- *Rhythm:* atrial—regular, ventricular—regular if block is constant; irregular if block is variable
- *Rate:* atrial—140 to 250 beats/minute, multiple of ventricular rate; ventricular—varies with block
- *P wave:* slightly abnormal
- *PR interval:* usually normal; may be hidden
- *QRS complex:* usually normal
- *Other:* more than one P wave for each QRS

(continued)

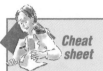

Identifying types of atrial tachycardia *(continued)*

Multifocal atrial tachycardia (MAT)

In MAT, atrial tachycardia occurs with numerous atrial foci firing intermittently. MAT produces varying P waves on the strip and occurs most commonly in patients with chronic pulmonary disease. The irregular baseline in this strip is caused by movement of the chest wall.

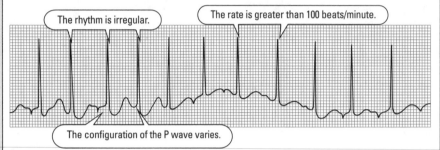

The rhythm is irregular.

The rate is greater than 100 beats/minute.

The configuration of the P wave varies.

Interpretation

• *Rhythm:* both irregular
• *Rate:* atrial — 100 to 250 beats/minute; usually under 160; ventricular — 100 to

250 beats/minute
• *P wave:* configuration varies; must see at least three different P wave

shapes
• *PR interval:* varies
• *Other:* none

Paroxysmal atrial tachycardia (PAT)

A type of paroxysmal supraventricular tachycardia (PSVT), PAT features brief periods of tachycardia that alternate with periods of normal sinus rhythm. PAT starts and stops suddenly as a result of rapid firing of an ectopic focus. It commonly follows frequent premature atrial contractions (PACs), one of which initiates the tachycardia.

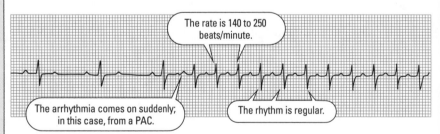

The rate is 140 to 250 beats/minute.

The arrhythmia comes on suddenly; in this case, from a PAC.

The rhythm is regular.

Interpretation

• *Rhythm:* regular
• *Rate:* 140 to 250 beats/minute
• *P wave:* abnormal, possibly

hidden in previous T wave
• *PR interval:* identical for each cycle
• *QRS complex:* can be aber-

rantly conducted
• *Other:* one P wave for each QRS complex

Indicators of atrial tachycardia

• *Atrial rhythm*—always regular
• *Ventricular rhythm*—regular when the block is constant and irregular when it isn't
• *Rate*—three or more successive ectopic atrial beats at a rate of 140 to 250 beats/minute; ventricular rate varies
• *P wave*—has a 1:1 ratio with QRS complex (unless a block is present); may not be discernible; may be hidden in previous ST segment or T wave
• *PR interval*—may not be able to measure
• *QRS complex*—usually normal
• *T wave*—normal or inverted
• *QT interval*—usually within normal limits; may be shorter
• *ST-segment and T-wave changes*—may appear if ischemia occurs

depending on the type of atrial tachycardia. A patient with paroxysmal atrial tachycardia may complain that his heart suddenly starts to beat faster or that he suddenly feels palpitations. Persistent tachycardia and rapid ventricular rate cause decreased cardiac output, which can lead to blurred vision, syncope, and hypotension.

How you intervene

Treatment depends on the type of tachycardia and the severity of the patient's symptoms. Because one of the most common causes

Understanding carotid sinus massage

Carotid sinus massage may be used to stop paroxysmal atrial tachycardia. Massaging the carotid sinus stimulates the vagus nerve, which then inhibits firing of the sinoatrial (SA) node and slows atrioventricular node conduction. As a result, the SA node can resume its job as primary pacemaker. Risks of carotid sinus massage include decreased heart rate, vasodilation, ventricular arrhythmias, cerebrovascular accident, and cardiac standstill.

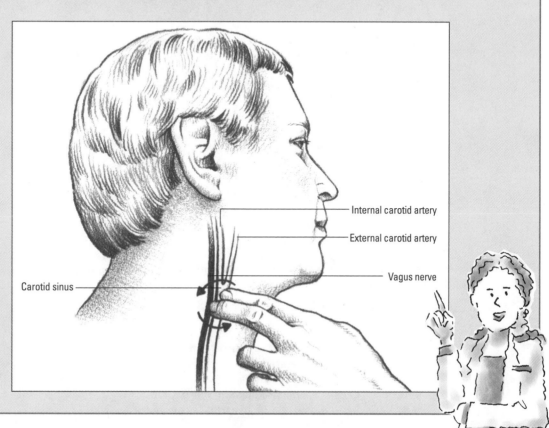

Internal carotid artery

External carotid artery

Vagus nerve

Carotid sinus

Atrial overdrive pacing

Atrial overdrive pacing (also called rapid atrial pacing) can stop atrial tachycardia. In this procedure, the patient's atrial rate is electronically paced slightly higher than the intrinsic atrial rate. With some patients, the atria are paced using much faster bursts or are paced prematurely at a critical time in the conduction cycle.

Whichever variation is used, the result is the same. The pacing interferes with the conduction circuit and renders part of it unresponsive to the reentrant impulse. Atrial tachycardia stops, and the sinoatrial node resumes its normal role as pacemaker.

of atrial tachycardia is digoxin toxicity, monitor levels of the drug. Measures to produce vagal stimulation, such as Valsalva's maneuver and carotid sinus massage, may be used to treat paroxysmal atrial tachycardia. (See *Understanding carotid sinus massage*, page 95.) These measures lead to slowing of the impulses from the SA and AV nodes, triggering atrial standstill and allowing the SA node to function as the primary pacemaker again.

Making a bigger block

A patient with atrial tachycardia can be given drugs that increase the degree of AV block, which in turn decreases the ventricular response and slows the rate. Such drugs include digoxin, beta-adrenergic blockers, and calcium channel blockers.

In addition, adenosine (Adenocard) can be used to stop atrial tachycardia, and quinidine (Cin-Quin) or procainamide (Pronestyl) can be used to establish normal sinus rhythm. When other treatments fail, synchronized cardioversion may be used. Atrial overdrive pacing (also called burst pacing) can be used to stop the arrhythmia. (See *Atrial overdrive pacing.*)

If the arrhythmia is associated with Wolff-Parkinson-White syndrome, catheter ablation (permanent damage of the area causing the arrhythmia) may be used to control recurrent episodes of paroxysmal atrial tachycardia. Because multifocal atrial tachycardia commonly occurs in patients with chronic obstructive pulmonary disease (COPD), the rhythm may not respond to treatment. Treatment attempts to correct severe hypoxia when possible.

Monitor the strip

When caring for a patient with atrial tachycardia, carefully monitor the patient's rhythm strips. Doing so may provide information about the cause of atrial tachycardia, which in turn can facilitate treatment.

Be alert to the possibility of digoxin toxicity. Frequent PACs may indicate that tachycardia is caused by reentry and therefore can be treated with a vagal maneuver. Remember that vagal stimulation can result in bradycardia, ventricular arrhythmias, and asystole. If vagal maneuvers are used, keep resuscitative equipment readily available.

Monitor the patient for chest pain, indications of decreased cardiac output, and signs and symptoms of heart failure or myocardial ischemia.

Atrial flutter

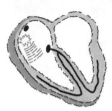

Atrial flutter, a supraventricular tachycardia, is characterized by an atrial rate of 250 to 400 beats/minute, although it's generally around 300 beats/minute. Originating in a single atrial focus, this rhythm results from circus reentry and possibly increased automaticity.

On an ECG, the P waves lose their distinction due to the rapid atrial rate. The waves blend together in a saw-tooth appearance and are called flutter waves, or *f* waves. These waves are the hallmark of atrial flutter.

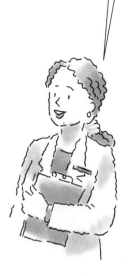

Atrial flutter often is associated with second-degree block.

How it happens

Atrial flutter is commonly associated with second-degree block. In that instance, the AV node fails to allow conduction of all the impulses to the ventricles. As a result, the ventricular rate is slower.

Atrial flutter may be caused by conditions that enlarge atrial tissue and elevate atrial pressures. It's commonly found in patients with severe mitral valve disease, hyperthyroidism, pericardial disease, and primary myocardial disease. The rhythm is also sometimes encountered in patients after cardiac surgery or in patients with acute MI, COPD, and systemic arterial hypoxia. Atrial flutter rarely occurs in a healthy person. When it does, it may indicate intrinsic cardiac disease.

Rating the ratio

The clinical significance of atrial flutter is determined by the number of impulses conducted through the node — expressed as a conduction ratio, for example, 2:1 or 4:1 — and the resulting ventricular rate. If the ventricular rate is too slow (fewer than 40 beats/minute) or too fast (more than 150 beats/minute), cardiac output can be seriously compromised.

Usually the faster the ventricular rate, the more dangerous the arrhythmia. The rapid rate reduces ventricular filling time and coronary perfusion, which can cause angina, heart failure, pulmonary edema, hypotension, and syncope.

What to look for

Atrial flutter is characterized by abnormal P waves that produce a saw-toothed appearance, the hallmark flutter-wave appearance. (See *Recognizing atrial flutter.*) Varying degrees of AV block produce ventricular rates one-half to one-fourth of the atrial rate.

The AV node usually won't accept more than 180 impulses/minute and allows every second, third, or fourth impulse to be conducted, the ratio of which determines the ventricular rate.

One of the most common rates is 150 beats/minute. With an atrial rate of 300, that rhythm is referred to as a 2:1 block. (See *Atrial flutter and sinus tachycardia.*)

The QRS complex is usually normal but may be widened if flutter waves are buried in the complex. You won't be able to identify a T wave, nor will you be able to measure the QT interval.

The atrial rhythm may vary between fibrillatory waves and flutter waves, an arrhythmia commonly referred to as atrial fibrillation and flutter.

Mixed signals

Atrial flutter and sinus tachycardia

Whenever you see sinus tachycardia with a rate of 150 beats/minute, take another look. That rate is a common one for atrial flutter with 2:1 conduction. Look closely for flutter waves, which may be difficult to see if they're hidden in the QRS complex. You may need to check another lead to clearly see them.

Recognizing atrial flutter

The following rhythm strip illustrates atrial flutter. Look for these distinguishing characteristics:

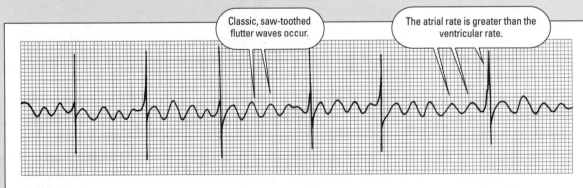

Classic, saw-toothed flutter waves occur.

The atrial rate is greater than the ventricular rate.

- *Rhythm:* atrial—regular; ventricular—irregular
- *Rate:* atrial—280 beats/minute; ventricular—60 beats/minute

- *P wave:* classic saw-toothed appearance
- *PR interval:* unmeasurable
- *QRS complex:* 0.08 second

- *T wave:* unidentifiable
- *QT interval:* unidentifiable
- *Other:* none.

Misleading pulses

When caring for a patient with atrial flutter, you may note that his peripheral or apical pulse is normal in rate and rhythm. That is because the pulse reflects the number of ventricular contractions, not the number of atrial impulses.

If the ventricular rate is normal, the patient may be asymptomatic. However, if the ventricular rate is rapid, the patient may exhibit signs and symptoms of reduced cardiac output and cardiac decompensation.

How you intervene

Atrial flutter with a rapid ventricular response and reduced cardiac output requires immediate intervention. Therapy aims to control the ventricular rate and convert the atrial ectopic rhythm to a normal sinus rhythm. Although stimulation of the vagus nerve may temporarily increase the block ratio and slow the ventricular rate, the effects won't last. For that reason, cardioversion remains the treatment of choice.

Synchronous shock

Synchronized cardioversion delivers an electrical stimulus during depolarization. The stimulus makes part of the myocardium refractory to ectopic impulses and terminates circus reentry movements.

Drug therapy includes digoxin and calcium channel blockers, which decrease AV conduction time. Quinidine may be given to convert flutter to fibrillation, an easier arrhythmia to treat. If digoxin and quinidine therapy is used, the patient must first be given a loading dose of digoxin. Ibutilide fumarate (Corvert) may be used to convert recent-onset atrial flutter to sinus rhythm. If possible, the underlying cause of the atrial flutter should be treated.

Stay alert

Because atrial flutter may be an indication of intrinsic cardiac disease, monitor the patient closely for signs and symptoms of low cardiac output. If cardioversion is indicated, prepare the patient for I.V. administration of a sedative or anesthetic as ordered. Keep resuscitative equipment at the bedside. Be alert to the effects of digoxin, which depresses the SA node. Also be alert for bradycardia. Cardioversion can decrease the heart rate.

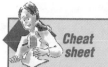

Cheat sheet

Indicators of atrial flutter

• *Rate*—atrial rate is usually greater than the ventricular rate
• *P waves*—abnormal with a saw-toothed appearance
• *QRS complex*—usually normal; may be widened if waves are buried in complex
• *T wave*—unidentifiable
• *QT interval*—unmeasurable

Atrial fibrillation

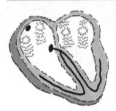

Atrial fibrillation, sometimes called "A-fib," is defined as chaotic, asynchronous, electrical activity in atrial tissue. It stems from the firing of a number of impulses in circus reentry pathways.

As with atrial flutter, atrial fibrillation results in a loss of atrial kick. The ectopic impulses may fire at a rate of 400 to 600 times/minute, causing the atria to quiver instead of contract.

The ventricles respond only to those impulses that make it through the AV node. On an ECG, atrial activity is no longer represented by P waves but by erratic baseline waves called fibrillatory waves, or f waves. This rhythm may be either sustained or paroxysmal (occurring in bursts). It can be either preceded by or be the result of PACs.

The irregular conduction of impulses through the AV node produces a characteristic irregularly irregular ventricular response. If you see R waves that look irregularly irregular, suspect atrial fibrillation.

How it happens

Atrial fibrillation occurs more commonly than atrial flutter or atrial tachycardia. Atrial fibrillation can occur following cardiac surgery, or it can be caused by mitral regurgitation, mitral stenosis, hyperthyroidism, infection, coronary artery disease, acute MI, pericarditis, hypoxia, and atrial septal defects.

The rhythm may also occur in a healthy person who uses coffee, alcohol, or cigarettes to excess or who is fatigued and under stress. Certain drugs, such as aminophylline and digoxin, may contribute to the development of atrial fibrillation. Catecholamine release during exercise may also trigger the arrhythmia.

Where have all the atrial kicks gone?

As with other atrial arrhythmias, atrial fibrillation eliminates atrial kick. That loss, combined with the decreased filling times associated with rapid rates, can lead to clinically significant problems. If the ventricular response is greater than 100 beats/minute — a condition called uncontrolled atrial fibrillation — the patient may develop heart failure, angina, or syncope.

Patients with preexisting cardiac disease, such as hypertrophic obstructive cardiomyopathy, mitral stenosis, rheumatic heart disease, and mitral prosthetic valves, tend to tolerate atrial fibrillation poorly and may develop shock and severe heart failure.

Risk of restoring sinus rhythm

A patient with atrial fibrillation is at increased risk for developing atrial thrombus and systemic arterial embolism. Because the atria don't contract, blood may pool on the atrial wall, and thrombi can form.

If normal sinus rhythm is restored and the atria contract normally, clots can break away and travel through the pulmonary or systemic circulation with potentially disastrous results.

Left untreated, atrial fibrillation can lead to cardiovascular collapse, thrombus formation, and systemic arterial or pulmonary embolism. (See *Risk of restoring sinus rhythm.*)

What to look for

Atrial fibrillation is distinguished by the absence of P waves and an irregular ventricular response. When a number of ectopic sites in the atria fire impulses, depolarization can't spread in an organized manner. (See *Recognizing atrial fibrillation.*)

Small sections of the atria are activated individually, which results in the atrial muscle quivering instead of contracting. On an ECG, you'll see uneven baseline f waves rather than clearly distinguishable P waves.

That fabulous filter

The AV node protects the ventricles from the 400 to 600 erratic atrial impulses that occur each minute by acting as a filter and blocking some of the impulses. The AV node itself doesn't receive all the impulses, however. If muscle tissue around the AV node is in a refractory state, impulses from other areas of the atria can't

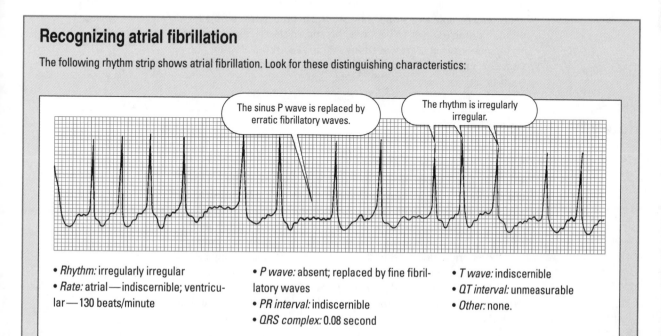

Recognizing atrial fibrillation

The following rhythm strip shows atrial fibrillation. Look for these distinguishing characteristics:

The sinus P wave is replaced by erratic fibrillatory waves.

The rhythm is irregularly irregular.

- *Rhythm:* irregularly irregular
- *Rate:* atrial—indiscernible; ventricular—130 beats/minute
- *P wave:* absent; replaced by fine fibrillatory waves
- *PR interval:* indiscernible
- *QRS complex:* 0.08 second
- *T wave:* indiscernible
- *QT interval:* unmeasurable
- *Other:* none.

reach the AV node, which further reduces the number of atrial impulses conducted through to the ventricles.

Those two factors help explain the characteristic wide variation in R-R intervals in atrial fibrillation.

Barely measurable

The atrial rate is almost indiscernible but is usually greater than 400 beats/minute. The ventricular rate usually varies from 100 to 150 beats/minute but can be lower. When the ventricular response rate is below 100, atrial fibrillation is considered controlled. When it exceeds 100, the rhythm is considered uncontrolled.

Atrial fibrillation is called coarse if the f waves are pronounced and fine if they aren't. Atrial fibrillation and flutter may also occur. Look for a configuration that varies between fibrillatory waves and flutter waves.

Pulse differences

When caring for a patient with atrial fibrillation, you may find that the radial pulse rate is slower than the apical rate. That is because unlike the stronger contractions, the weaker contractions of the heart don't produce a palpable peripheral pulse.

The pulse rhythm will be irregular. If the ventricular rate is rapid, the patient may show signs and symptoms of decreased cardiac output, including hypotension and light-headedness. His heart may be able to compensate for the decrease if the fibrillation lasts long enough to become chronic. In those cases, however, the patient is at a greater-than-normal risk of developing pulmonary, cerebral, or other emboli and may exhibit signs of those conditions.

How you intervene

The major therapeutic goal in treating atrial fibrillation is to reduce the ventricular response rate to below 100 beats/minute. This may be accomplished either by drugs that control the ventricular response or by cardioversion and drugs in combination to convert the rhythm to sinus.

The ventricular rate may be controlled with such drugs as diltiazem (Cardizem), verapamil (Isoptin), digoxin (Lanoxin), and beta-adrenergic blockers. Ibutilide fumarate (Corvert) may be used to convert new-onset atrial fibrillation to sinus rhythm. Quinidine (Cin-Quin) and procainamide (Pronestyl) can also convert atrial fibrillation to normal sinus rhythm, usually after anticoagulation.

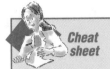

Cheat sheet

Indicators of atrial fibrillation

- *Atrial rate*—usually greater than 400 beats/minute
- *P waves*—absent
- *Ventricular response*—irregular; varies from 100 to 150 beats/minute but can be lower
- *f waves*—seen as uneven baseline on ECG rather than distinguishable P waves
- *R-R intervals*—wide variation

Three critical days

Electrical cardioversion is most successful if used within the first 3 days of treatment and less successful if the rhythm has existed for a long time. If the patient shows signs of more severe angina or of decreased cardiac output, emergency measures are necessary.

When the onset of atrial fibrillation is acute and the patient can cooperate, vagal maneuvers or carotid sinus massage may slow the ventricular response but won't convert the arrhythmia.

Cardioversion

A symptomatic patient needs immediate synchronized cardioversion. If possible, anticoagulants should be administered first because cardioversion can cause emboli to form, especially in patients with chronic or paroxysmal atrial fibrillation.

A conversion to normal sinus rhythm will cause forceful atrial contractions to resume abruptly. If a thrombus forms in the atria, the resumption of contractions can result in systemic emboli. (See *How synchronized cardioversion works.*)

Reestablishing its role

Drugs such as digoxin, procainamide, propranolol (Inderal), quinidine, amiodarone, and verapamil can be given after successful cardioversion to maintain normal sinus rhythm and to control the ventricular rate in chronic atrial fibrillation. Some of these drugs

---

How synchronized cardioversion works

A patient whose arrhythmia causes low cardiac output and hypotension may be a candidate for synchronized cardioversion. This may be an elective or emergency procedure. For instance, it may be used to make a person with atrial fibrillation more comfortable or to save the life of a patient with ventricular tachycardia.

Synchronize the energy
Synchronized cardioversion is similar to defibrillation except that cardioversion generally requires lower energy levels. In synchronized cardioversion, the R wave on the patient's electrocardiogram is synchronized with the cardioverter (defibrillator). After the firing buttons have been pressed, the cardioverter discharges energy when it senses the next R wave.

When the stimulus hits
To stop atrial depolarization and reestablish normal sinus rhythm, stimulation must occur during the R wave. Stimulation that hits a T wave increases the risk of fatal arrhythmias. Keep in mind that there is a slight delay between the time the firing button is pressed and the moment the energy is actually discharged. Hold the paddles to the patient's chest until the energy is actually discharged.

Use in digoxin toxicity
Be aware that synchronized cardioversion carries the risk of lethal arrhythmias when used in patients with digoxin toxicity.

prolong the atrial refractory period, giving the SA node an opportunity to reestablish its role as the heart's pacemaker, whereas others primarily slow AV node conduction, controlling the ventricular rate. Symptomatic atrial fibrillation that doesn't respond to routine treatment may be treated with radiofrequency ablation therapy.

When assessing a patient with atrial fibrillation, assess both the peripheral and apical pulses. If the patient isn't on a cardiac monitor, be alert for an irregular pulse and differences in the apical and radial pulse rates.

Assess for symptoms of decreased cardiac output and heart failure. If drug therapy is used, monitor serum drug levels and observe the patient for evidence of toxicity. Tell the patient to report pulse rate changes, syncope or dizziness, chest pain, or signs of heart failure, such as increasing dyspnea and peripheral edema.

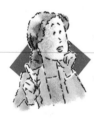

Quick quiz

1. The hallmark of a premature atrial contraction is a:
    A. regular atrial rhythm.
    B. premature, abnormally shaped P wave.
    C. P wave followed by an aberrantly conducted QRS complex.

Answer: B. Because PACs originate outside the SA node, the P wave comes earlier in the cycle and has a different configuration than the sinus P wave.

2. In atrial flutter, the key consideration in determining treatment is the:
    A. atrial rate.
    B. ventricular rate.
    C. configuration of the flutter waves.

Answer: B. If the ventricular rate is too fast or too slow, cardiac output will be compromised. A rapid ventricular rate may require immediate cardioversion.

3. In controlled atrial fibrillation, the ventricular response rate is:
    A. lower than 60 beats/minute.
    B. lower than 100 beats/minute.
    C. higher than 100 beats/minute.

Answer: B. Atrial fibrillation with a ventricular response rate lower than 100 is considered controlled and commonly requires no treatment. A rate above 100 is considered uncontrolled and may require cardioversion or other treatment.

4. Carotid sinus massage is used to:
   A. prevent the continued development of PACs.
   B. increase the ventricular rate in AV block.
   C. convert paroxysmal atrial tachycardia to sinus rhythm.

Answer: C. Carotid sinus massage triggers atrial standstill by inhibiting firing of the SA node and slowing AV conduction. This allows the SA node to reestablish itself as the primary pacemaker. In atrial flutter, the technique may increase the block and slow the ventricular rate but won't convert the rhythm.

5. For atrial fibrillation, electrical cardioversion is most successful if used:
   A. during the first 3 days after the onset of the arrhythmia.
   B. during the first 3 weeks of treatment for the arrhythmia.
   C. during the first 3 months after the onset of the arrhythmia.

Answer: A. Electrical cardioversion is most successful if used within the first 3 days of treatment and less successful if the rhythm has existed for a long time.

Test strips

Try a couple of test strips. Answer the questions accompanying each strip; then check your answers with ours.

6. In the strip shown below, the rhythm is regular, the atrial rate is 310 beats/minute, the ventricular rate is 80 beats/minute, the P wave consists of saw-tooth-shaped waves, the PR interval is unmeasurable, the QRS complex is 0.08 second, the T wave is unidentifiable, and the QT interval is unmeasurable. You would identify the strip as:
   A. atrial tachycardia.
   B. atrial fibrillation.
   C. atrial flutter.

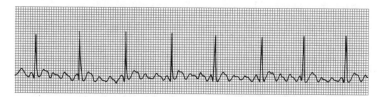

Answer: C. The characteristic saw-toothed appearance of the P waves is a classic indication of atrial flutter.

7. In the ECG strip shown below, the rhythm is irregular, the rate is 80 beats/minute, the P wave is normal, the PR interval is 0.14 second, the QRS complex is 0.08 second, the T wave is normal, and the QT interval is 0.36 second. You would identify the strip as:

    A.   atrial fibrillation.
    B.   atrial tachycardia.
    C.   normal sinus rhythm with PACs.

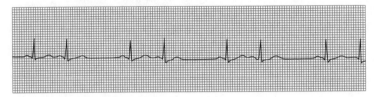

Answer: C. This is normal sinus rhythm with PACs occurring after each sinus beat.

8. You notice the following rhythm on the monitor and obtain a rhythm strip. After examining the characteristics of the strip, you identify the rhythm as:

    A.   atrial fibrillation.
    B.   atrial tachycardia.
    C.   normal sinus rhythm with PACs.

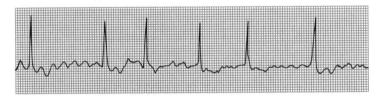

Answer: A. This is coarse atrial fibrillation with aberrant ventricular conduction. The rhythm is irregular, the atrial rate can't be determined, the ventricular rate is 60 beats/minute, the P wave is absent, coarse fibrillatory waves are present, the PR interval is indiscernible, the duration of the QRS complex is 0.12 second, the T wave is indiscernible, and the QT interval is unmeasurable.

Scoring

☆☆☆ If you answered all eight questions correctly, outstanding! You're the MVP of the Atrial World Series!

☆☆ If you answered five to seven questions correctly, super! You're an up-and-coming power hitter, destined for the Atrial Hall of Fame!

☆ If you answered fewer than five questions correctly, hang in there. With a little batting practice, you'll be smacking home runs at Atrial Park in no time!

Junctional arrhythmias

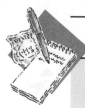

Just the facts

This chapter describes the various types of junctional arrhythmias and how they're treated. In this chapter, you'll learn:

♦ the characteristics of junctional arrhythmias

♦ the causes of junctional arrhythmias and which patients are at risk for them

♦ how junctional arrhythmias look on an ECG strip

♦ what assessment findings are associated with certain arrhythmias

♦ how to treat junctional arrhythmias and care for patients who have them.

A look at junctional arrhythmias

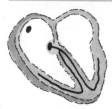

Junctional arrhythmias originate in the atrioventricular (AV) junction—the area around the AV node and the bundle of His. The arrhythmias occur when the sinoatrial (SA) node, a higher pacemaker, is suppressed and fails to conduct impulses or when a block occurs in conduction. Electrical impulses may then be initiated by pacemaker cells in the AV junction.

Just your normal impulse

In normal impulse conduction, the AV node slows transmission of the impulse from the atria to the ventricles, which allows the atria to pump as much blood as they can into the ventricles before the ventricles contract. But impulses aren't always conducted normally. (See *Conduction in Wolff-Parkinson-White syndrome,* page 108.)

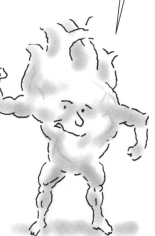

Normal impulses keep the blood pumping.

Now I get it!

Conduction in Wolff-Parkinson-White syndrome

Conduction doesn't always take place in a normal way. In Wolff-Parkinson-White syndrome, for example, a conduction bypass develops outside the atrioventricular (AV) junction and connects the atria with the ventricles, as shown. Wolff-Parkinson-White syndrome is typically a congenital rhythm disorder that occurs mainly in young children and in adults ages 20 to 35.

Rapidly conducted
The bypass formed in Wolff-Parkinson-White syndrome, known as the bundle of Kent, conducts impulses to the atria or the ventricles. Impulses aren't delayed at the AV node, so conduction is abnormally fast. Retrograde conduction, circus reentry, and reentrant tachycardia can result.

Checking the ECG
This syndrome causes a shortened PR interval (less than 0.10 second) and a widened QRS complex (greater than 0.10 second). The beginning of the QRS complex may look slurred because of altered ventricular depolarization. This hallmark sign of Wolff-Parkinson-White syndrome is called a delta wave, shown in the inset.

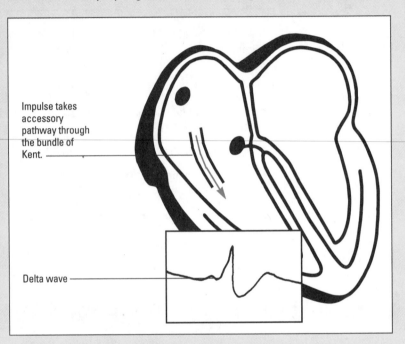

Impulse takes accessory pathway through the bundle of Kent.

Delta wave

Because the AV junction is located in the middle of the heart, impulses generated in this area cause the heart to be depolarized in an abnormal way. The impulse moves upward and causes backward, or retrograde, depolarization of the atria and inverted P waves in leads II, III, and aV$_F$, leads in which you would normally see upright P waves. (See *Finding the P wave.*)

Which way did the impulse go?

The impulse also moves down toward the ventricles, causing forward, or antegrade, depolarization of the ventricles and an upright QRS complex. Arrhythmias that cause inverted P waves on an electrocardiogram (ECG) may be atrial or junctional in origin.

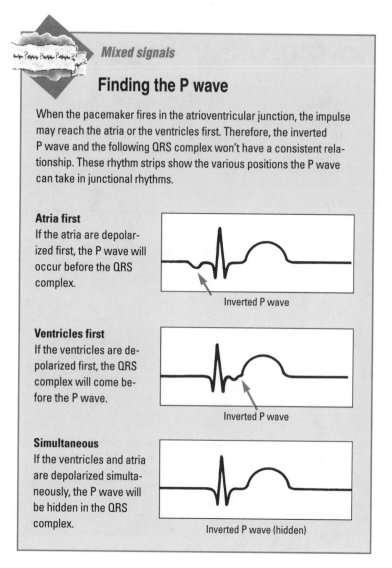

Mixed signals

Finding the P wave

When the pacemaker fires in the atrioventricular junction, the impulse may reach the atria or the ventricles first. Therefore, the inverted P wave and the following QRS complex won't have a consistent relationship. These rhythm strips show the various positions the P wave can take in junctional rhythms.

Atria first
If the atria are depolarized first, the P wave will occur before the QRS complex.

Inverted P wave

Ventricles first
If the ventricles are depolarized first, the QRS complex will come before the P wave.

Inverted P wave

Simultaneous
If the ventricles and atria are depolarized simultaneously, the P wave will be hidden in the QRS complex.

Inverted P wave (hidden)

Junctional mimic

Atrial arrhythmias are sometimes mistaken for junctional arrhythmias because impulses are generated so low in the atria that they cause retrograde depolarization and inverted P waves. Looking at the PR interval will help you determine whether an arrhythmia is atrial or junctional.

An arrhythmia with an inverted P wave before the QRS complex and a normal PR interval (0.12 to 0.20 second) originated in the atria. An arrhythmia with a PR interval less than 0.12 second originated in the AV junction.

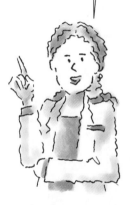

Don't mistake an atrial arrhythmia for a junctional arrhythmia. Check the PR interval.

Premature junctional contraction

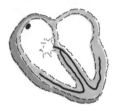

A premature junctional contraction (PJC) is a beat that occurs before a normal beat and causes an irregular rhythm. This ectopic beat occurs when an irritable location within the AV junction acts as a pacemaker and fires either prematurely or out of sequence.

As with all beats produced by the AV junction, the atria are depolarized in retrograde fashion, causing an inverted P wave. The ventricles are depolarized normally.

How it happens

PJCs may be caused by toxic levels of digoxin (level greater than 2.5 ng/ml), excessive caffeine intake, inferior-wall myocardial infarction (MI), rheumatic heart disease, valvular disease, or swelling of the AV junction after heart surgery.

The beat goes on

Although PJCs themselves usually aren't dangerous, you'll need to monitor the patient carefully and assess him for other signs of intrinsic pacemaker failure.

What to look for

A PJC appears on a rhythm strip as an early beat causing an irregularity. The rest of the strip may show regular atrial and ventricular rhythms, depending on the patient's underlying rhythm.

P wave inversion

Look for an inverted P wave in leads II, III, and aV_F. Depending on when the impulse occurs, the P wave may fall before, during, or after the QRS complex. (See *Identifying a PJC*.) If it falls during the QRS complex, it's hidden. If it comes before the QRS complex, the PR interval is less than 0.12 second.

Because the ventricles are usually depolarized normally, the QRS complex has a normal configuration and a normal duration of less than 0.12 second. The T wave and the QT interval are usually normal.

That quickening feeling

The patient may be asymptomatic or he may complain of palpitations or a feeling of quickening in the chest. You may be able to palpate an irregular pulse. If the PJCs are frequent enough, the pa-

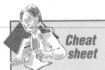

Cheat sheet

Recognizing a PJC

- *Rhythm:* irregular with PJC appearance
- *Rate:* varies with underlying rhythm
- *P wave:* inverted; falls before or after or is hidden in QRS complex; may be absent
- *PR interval:* less than 0.12 second or unmeasurable
- *QRS complex:* usually normal
- *T wave:* usually normal
- *QT interval:* usually normal
- *Other:* noncompensatory pause after PJC

Identifying a PJC

This ECG strip shows a premature junctional contraction (PJC)—a junctional beat that occurs before a normal sinus beat.

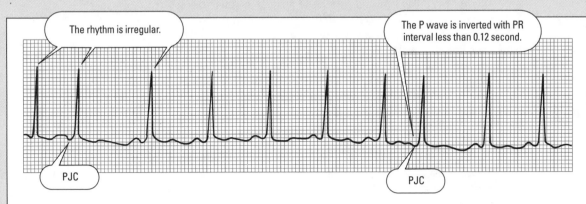

The rhythm is irregular.

The P wave is inverted with PR interval less than 0.12 second.

PJC

PJC

- *Rhythm:* irregular atrial and ventricular rhythms
- *Rate:* 100 beats/minute
- *P wave:* inverted and precedes the QRS complex

- *PR interval:* 0.14 second for the underlying rhythm and 0.06 second for the PJC

- *QRS complex:* 0.06 second
- *T wave:* normal configuration
- *QT interval:* 0.36 second
- *Other:* pause after PJC

tient may have hypotension from a transient decrease in cardiac output.

How you intervene

PJCs usually don't require treatment unless symptoms occur. In those cases, the underlying cause should be treated. If digoxin toxicity is the culprit, the medication should be discontinued and serum drug levels monitored.

You should also monitor the patient for hemodynamic instability. If ectopic beats are frequent, the patient should decrease or eliminate his caffeine intake.

Junctional escape rhythm

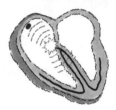

A junctional escape rhythm is a string of beats that occurs after a conduction delay from the atria. The normal intrinsic firing rate for cells in the AV junction is 40 to 60 beats/minute.

Remember that the AV junction can take over as the heart's pacemaker if higher pacemaker sites slow down or fail to fire or conduct. The junctional escape beat is an example of this compensatory mechanism. Because junctional escape beats prevent ventricular standstill, they should never be suppressed.

Backward and upside-down

In a junctional escape rhythm, as in all junctional arrhythmias, the atria are depolarized by means of retrograde conduction. The P waves are inverted, and impulse conduction through the ventricles is normal.

How it happens

A junctional escape rhythm can be caused by any condition that disturbs SA node function or enhances AV junction automaticity. Causes of the arrhythmia include:
- sick sinus syndrome
- vagal stimulation
- digoxin toxicity
- inferior-wall MI
- rheumatic heart disease.

The great escape

Whether junctional escape rhythm harms the patient depends on how well the patient's heart tolerates a decreased heart rate and decreased cardiac output. The less tolerant the heart is, the more significant the effects of the arrhythmia.

What to look for

A junctional escape rhythm shows a regular rhythm of 40 to 60 beats/minute on an ECG strip. Look for inverted P waves in leads II, III, and aV$_F$.

The P waves will occur before, after, or hidden within the QRS complex. The PR interval is less than 0.12 second and is measurable only if the P wave comes before the QRS complex. (See *Identifying junctional escape rhythm.*)

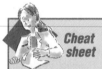

Cheat sheet

Recognizing junctional escape rhythm

- *Rhythm:* regular
- *Rate:* 40 to 60 beats/ minute
- *P wave:* inverted in leads II, III, and aV$_F$; can occur before, during, or after the QRS complex
- *PR interval:* less than 0.12 second if the P wave comes before the QRS complex
- *QRS complex:* normal; less than 0.12 second
- *T wave:* normal
- *QT interval:* normal
- *Other:* none

Don't skip this strip

Identifying junctional escape rhythm

This ECG strip shows a junctional escape rhythm. Note the inverted P wave.

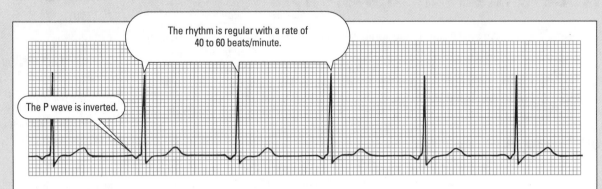

The rhythm is regular with a rate of 40 to 60 beats/minute.

The P wave is inverted.

- *Rhythm:* regular
- *Rate:* 60 beats/minute
- *P wave:* inverted and preceding each QRS complex

- *PR interval:* 0.10 second
- *QRS complex:* 0.10 second
- *T wave:* normal

- *QT interval:* 0.44 second
- *Other:* none

The rest of the ECG waveform — including the QRS complex, T wave, and QT interval — should appear normal because impulses through the ventricles are usually conducted normally.

I may be slow, but at least I'm regular

A patient with a junctional escape rhythm will have a slow, regular pulse rate of 40 to 60 beats/minute. The patient may be asymptomatic. However, pulse rates less than 60 beats/minute may lead to inadequate cardiac output, causing hypotension, syncope, or blurred vision.

How you intervene

Treatment for a junctional escape rhythm involves correcting the underlying cause. Atropine may be given to increase the heart rate, or a temporary or permanent pacemaker may be inserted. (See *Treatment of junctional escape rhythm.*)

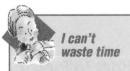

I can't waste time

Treatment of junctional escape rhythm

- Correct the underlying cause.
- Atropine may be given.
- A temporary or permanent pacemaker may be inserted.

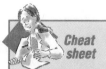

Nursing care includes monitoring the patient's serum digoxin and electrolyte levels and watching for signs of decreased cardiac output, such as hypotension, syncope, or blurred vision. If the patient is hypotensive, lower the head of his bed as far as he can tolerate it and keep atropine at the bedside.

Accelerated junctional rhythm

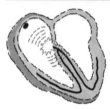

An accelerated junctional rhythm is caused by an irritable focus in the AV junction that speeds up to take over as the heart's pacemaker. The atria are depolarized by means of retrograde conduction, and the ventricles are depolarized normally. The accelerated rate is usually between 60 and 100 beats/minute.

How it happens

Conditions that affect SA node or AV node automaticity can cause accelerated junctional rhythm. Those conditions include:
- digoxin toxicity
- hypokalemia
- inferior- or posterior-wall MI
- rheumatic heart disease
- valvular heart disease.

Getting a kick out of it

This arrhythmia is significant if the patient has symptoms of decreased cardiac output — hypotension, syncope, and blurred vision. These can occur if the atria are depolarized after the QRS complex, which prevents blood ejection from the atria into the ventricles, or atrial kick.

What to look for

With an accelerated junctional rhythm, look for a regular rhythm and a rate of 60 to 100 beats/minute. (See *Identifying accelerated junctional rhythm.*) If the P wave is present, it will be inverted in leads II, III, and aV$_F$ and will occur before or after the QRS complex or be hidden in it. If the P wave comes before the QRS complex, the PR interval will be less than 0.12 second. The QRS complex, T wave, and QT interval all appear normal.

Cheat sheet

Recognizing accelerated junctional rhythm

- *Rhythm:* regular
- *Rate:* 60 to 100 beats/minute
- *P wave:* inverted in leads II, III and aV$_F$ (if present) and occurring before, during, or after QRS complex
- *PR interval:* measurable only with P wave that comes before QRS complex; 0.12 second or less
- *QRS complex:* usually normal
- *T wave:* usually normal
- *QT interval:* usually normal
- *Other:* none

Look for a regular rhythm.

Identifying accelerated junctional rhythm

This ECG strip shows an accelerated junctional rhythm.

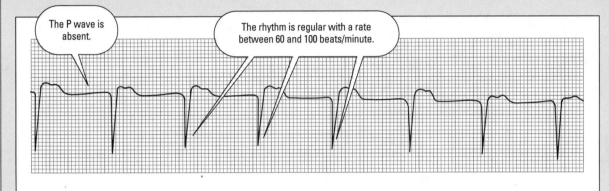

The P wave is absent.

The rhythm is regular with a rate between 60 and 100 beats/minute.

- *Rhythm:* regular
- *Rate:* 80 beats/minute
- *P wave:* absent
- *PR interval:* unmeasurable

- *QRS complex:* 0.10 second
- *T wave:* normal
- *QT interval:* 0.32 second
- *Other:* none

Low-down, dizzy, and confused

The patient may be asymptomatic because accelerated junctional rhythm has the same rate as sinus rhythm. However, if cardiac output is low, the patient may become dizzy, hypotensive, and confused and have weak peripheral pulses.

How you intervene

Treatment for accelerated junctional arrhythmia involves correcting the underlying cause. Nursing interventions include observing the patient to see how well he tolerates this arrhythmia, monitoring his digoxin level, and withholding his digoxin dose as ordered.

You should also assess the levels of potassium and other electrolytes and administer supplements as ordered; monitor vital signs for hemodynamic instability; and observe for signs of decreased cardiac output.

Junctional tachycardia

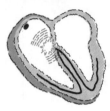

In junctional tachycardia, three or more premature junctional contractions occur in a row. This supraventricular tachycardia occurs when an irritable focus from the AV junction has enhanced automaticity, overriding the SA node to function as the heart's pacemaker.

In this arrhythmia, the atria are depolarized by means of retrograde conduction, and conduction through the ventricles is normal. The rate is usually 100 to 200 beats/minute. (See *Identifying junctional tachycardia.*)

How it happens

Possible causes of junctional tachycardia include:
• digoxin toxicity (most common cause), which can be enhanced by hypokalemia
• inferior- or posterior-wall MI or ischemia

Identifying junctional tachycardia

This ECG strip shows junctional tachycardia.

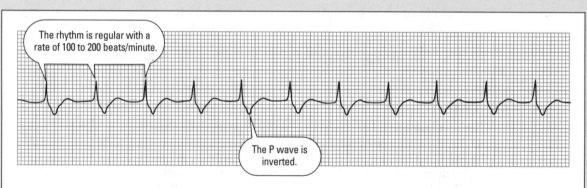

The rhythm is regular with a rate of 100 to 200 beats/minute.

The P wave is inverted.

• *Rhythm:* regular atrial and ventricular rhythms
• *Rate:* atrial and ventricular rates of 115 beats/minute

• *P wave:* inverted, follows QRS complex
• *PR interval:* unmeasurable
• *QRS complex:* 0.08 second

• *T wave:* normal
• *QT interval:* 0.36 second
• *Other:* none

- congenital heart disease in children
- swelling of the AV junction after heart surgery.

Compromisin' rhythm

The significance of junctional tachycardia depends on the rate, underlying cause, and severity of the accompanying cardiac disease. At higher ventricular rates, junctional tachycardia may compromise cardiac output by decreasing the amount of blood filling the ventricles with each beat. Higher rates also result in the loss of atrial kick.

What to look for

When assessing a rhythm strip for junctional tachycardia, look for a rate of 100 to 200 beats/minute. The P wave is inverted in leads II, III, and aV_F and can occur before, during (hidden P wave), or after the QRS complex.

Measurement of the PR interval depends on whether the P wave falls before, in, or after the QRS complex. If it comes before the QRS complex, the only time the PR interval can be measured, it will always be less than 0.12 second.

The QRS complexes look normal, as does the T wave, unless a P wave occurs in it or the rate is so fast that the T wave can't be detected. (See *Junctional and supraventricular tachycardia*.)

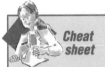

Cheat sheet

Recognizing junctional tachycardia

- *Rhythm:* regular
- *Rate:* 100 to 200 beats/minute
- *P wave:* inverted in leads II, III and aV_F; location varies around QRS complex
- *PR interval:* shortened at less than 0.12 second or unmeasurable
- *QRS complex:* normal
- *T wave:* usually normal but may contain P wave
- *QT interval:* usually normal
- *Other:* none

Mixed signals

Junctional and supraventricular tachycardia

If a tachycardia has a narrow QRS complex, you may have trouble deciding whether its source is junctional or atrial. Once the rate approaches 150 beats/minute, a formerly visible P wave is hidden in the previous T wave, so you won't be able to use the P wave to figure out where the rhythm originated.

In these cases, call the rhythm *supraventricular* tachycardia, a general term that refers to the origin as being above the ventricles. Examples of supraventricular tachycardia include atrial flutter, multifocal atrial tachycardia, and junctional tachycardia.

Rapid rate = instability

Patients with rapid heart rates may have decreased cardiac output and hemodynamic instability. The pulse will be rapid, and dizziness, low blood pressure, and other signs of decreased cardiac output may be present.

How you intervene

The underlying cause should be treated. If the cause is digoxin toxicity, the digoxin should be discontinued. Vagal maneuvers and medications such as verapamil may slow the heart rate for the symptomatic patient. (See *Comparing junctional rates.*)

If the patient recently had an MI or heart surgery, he may need a temporary pacemaker to reset the heart's rhythm. Children with permanent arrhythmias may be resistant to drug therapy and require surgery. Patients with recurrent junctional tachycardia may be treated with ablation therapy, followed by permanent pacemaker insertion.

Monitor patients with junctional tachycardia for signs of decreased cardiac output. You should also check digoxin and potassium levels and administer potassium supplements, as ordered. If symptoms are severe and digoxin is the culprit, the doctor may order Digibind, a digoxin-binding drug.

Comparing junctional rates

The names given to junctional rhythms vary according to rate. The illustration below shows how each rhythm's name and rate are correlated.

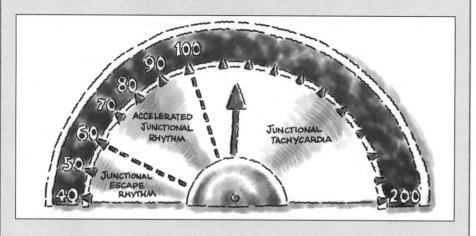

Wandering pacemaker

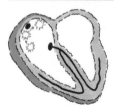

A wandering pacemaker is an irregular rhythm that results when the heart's pacemaker changes its focus from the SA node to another area above the ventricles. The origin of the impulse may wander beat-to-beat from the SA node to other atrial sites or to the AV junction. The P wave and PR interval vary from beat to beat as the pacemaker site changes. (See *Key facts about wandering pacemaker*.)

How it happens

Wandering pacemaker may be caused by:
• increased vagal tone
• digoxin toxicity
• organic heart disease, such as rheumatic carditis.

The arrhythmia may be normal in young patients and is common in athletes who have slow heart rates. It may be difficult to identify because the arrhythmia is often transient. Although wandering pacemaker is rarely serious, chronic arrhythmias are a sign of heart disease and should be monitored.

What to look for

The rhythm on an ECG strip will look slightly irregular because sites of impulse initiation vary. The rate is usually normal — 60 to 100 beats/minute — but it may be slower. The P waves change shape as the pacemaker site changes.

Impulses may originate in the SA node, atria, or AV junction. If an impulse originates in the AV junction, the P wave may come before, during, or after the QRS complex. The PR interval will also vary from beat to beat as the pacemaker site changes, but it will always be less than 0.20 second.

Mind the PRs and QRSs

The variation in PR interval will cause a slightly irregular R-R interval. If the impulse originates in the AV junction, the PR interval will be less than 0.12 second. Ventricular depolarization is normal, so the QRS complex will be less than 0.12 second. The T wave and QT interval will usually be normal, although the QT interval can vary. (See *Identifying wandering pacemaker*, page 120.)

Patients are generally asymptomatic and unaware of the arrhythmia. The pulse rate and rhythm may be normal or irregular.

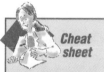

Cheat sheet

Recognizing wandering pacemaker

• *Rhythm:* irregular
• *Rate:* usually normal or below 60 beats/ minute
• *P wave:* changes in size and shape
• *PR interval:* varies
• *QRS complex:* usually normal
• *T wave:* normal
• *QT interval:* may vary
• *Other:* none

Key facts about wandering pacemaker

• The name of this arrhythmia suggests its nature. The origins of the impulses wander around the atria and atrioventricular junction.
• You'll see varying P waves on the ECG strip.
• This arrhythmia usually is transient and benign and is common in young children and athletes.

Identifying wandering pacemaker

This ECG strip shows wandering pacemaker—an atrial arrhythmia with a shifting impulse site. Note the difference in P waves caused by those impulse shifts.

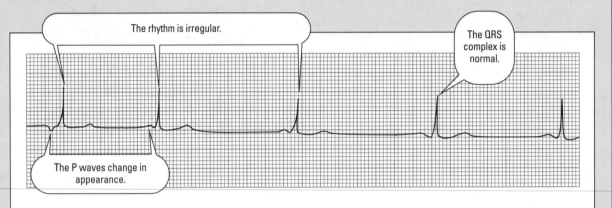

The rhythm is irregular.

The QRS complex is normal.

The P waves change in appearance.

- *Rhythm:* irregular atrial and ventricular rhythms
- *Rate:* atrial and ventricular rates are 50 beats/minute

- *P wave:* changes in size and shape; first P wave is inverted, second is upright
- *PR interval:* varies

- *QRS complex:* 0.08 second
- *T wave:* normal
- *QT interval:* 0.44 second
- *Other:* none

How you intervene

Usually, no treatment is needed. If the patient is symptomatic, however, the underlying cause should be treated.

You'll need to monitor the patient's heart rhythm and assess for signs of hemodynamic instability. Also assess blood pressure, mental status, and skin color.

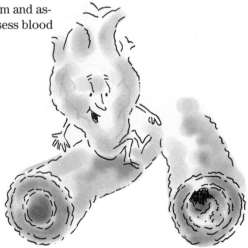

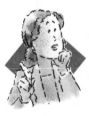

Quick quiz

1. In a junctional escape rhythm, the P wave can occur:
   A.   within the T wave.
   B.   on top of the preceding Q wave.
   C.   before, during, or after the QRS complex.

Answer: C. In all junctional arrhythmias, the P wave is inverted in leads II, III, and aV$_F$ and may appear before, during, or after the QRS complex.

2. In an accelerated junctional rhythm, the QRS complex appears:
   A.   narrowed.
   B.   widened.
   C.   normal.

Answer: C. Because the ventricles are usually depolarized normally in this rhythm, the QRS complex has a normal configuration and a normal duration of less than 0.12 second.

3. The normal slowing of impulses as they pass through the AV node allows the atria to:
   A.   fill completely with blood from the venae cavae.
   B.   pump the maximum amount of blood possible into the ventricles.
   C.   remain insensitive to ectopic impulse formation outside the sinus node.

Answer: B. In normal impulse conduction, the AV node slows impulse transmission from the atria to the ventricles and allows the atria to pump as much blood as possible into the ventricles before the ventricles contract.

4. If the ventricles are depolarized first in a junctional rhythm, the P wave will appear:
   A.   before the QRS complex.
   B.   within the QRS complex.
   C.   after the QRS complex.

Answer: C. If the ventricles are depolarized first, the P wave will come after the QRS complex.

Test strips

Following are two test strips. Answer the question accompanying each strip; then check your answers with ours.

5. Below, atrial and ventricular rhythms are regular at 47 beats/minute, P wave is inverted, PR interval is 0.08 second, QRS complex is 0.06 second, T wave is normal, and QT interval is 0.42 second. You would interpret this rhythm as:

    A.   wandering pacemaker.
    B.   junctional tachycardia.
    C.   junctional escape rhythm.

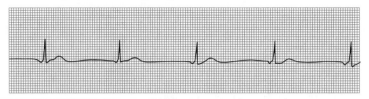

Answer: C. This strip shows junctional escape rhythm.

6. You would interpret the rhythm shown below as:

    A.   junctional escape rhythm.
    B.   junctional tachycardia.
    C.   sinus bradycardia with a PJC.

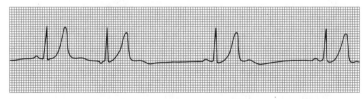

Answer: B. Atrial and ventricular rhythms are irregular at 40 beats/minute, P wave occurs on the second beat, PR interval is 0.08 on second beat and 0.16 second on others, QRS complex is 0.08 second, T wave is tall and peaked, and QT interval is 0.48 second. These observations indicate sinus bradycardia with a PJC.

Scoring

☆☆☆ If you answered all six questions correctly, we're impressed! Dance away to that hot new band, the Junctional Escape Rhythms!

☆☆ If you answered four to five questions correctly, wow! You've clearly got that accelerated junctional rhythm!

☆ If you answered fewer than four questions correctly, we still think your heart is in the right place!

Ventricular arrhythmias

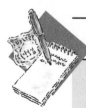

Just the facts

This chapter discusses the types of ventricular arrhythmias and how each is treated. In this chapter, you'll learn:

♦ where ventricular arrhythmias originate

♦ what characterizes each ventricular arrhythmia

♦ what causes ventricular arrhythmias and which patients are at risk for developing them

♦ how to interpret ventricular arrhythmias on an electrocardiogram strip

♦ how to treat, assess, and care for a patient with a ventricular arrhythmia.

A look at ventricular arrhythmias

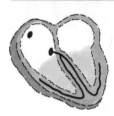

Ventricular arrhythmias originate in the ventricles below the bundle of His. They occur when electrical impulses depolarize the myocardium using a different pathway from normal impulses.

Ventricular arrhythmias appear on an electrocardiogram (ECG) in characteristic ways. The QRS complex is wider than normal because of the prolonged conduction time through the ventricles. The T wave and the QRS complex deflect in opposite directions because of the difference in the action potential during ventricular depolarization and repolarization. Also, the P wave is absent because atrial depolarization doesn't occur.

No kick from the atria

When electrical impulses are generated from the ventricles instead of the atria, atrial kick is lost and cardiac output decreases by as much as 30%. As a result, patients with ventricular arrhythmias may show signs and symptoms of cardiac decompensation, including hypotension, angina, syncope, and respiratory distress.

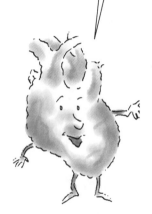

Ventricular arrhythmias appear on an ECG in characteristic ways.

Potential to kill

Although ventricular arrhythmias may be benign, they're potentially deadly because the ventricles are ultimately responsible for cardiac output. Rapid recognition and treatment of ventricular arrhythmias increases the chance for successful resuscitation.

Premature ventricular contraction

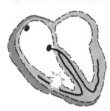

A premature ventricular contraction (PVC) is an ectopic beat that may occur in healthy people without causing problems. PVCs may occur singly, in clusters of two or more, or in repeating patterns, such as bigeminy or trigeminy. (See *Identifying PVCs.*) When PVCs occur in patients with underlying heart disease, they may indicate impending lethal ventricular arrhythmias.

How it happens

PVCs are usually caused by electrical irritability in the ventricular conduction system or muscle tissue. This irritability may be provoked by anything that disrupts normal electrolyte shifts during cell depolarization and repolarization. Conditions that can disrupt electrolyte shifts include:
- electrolyte imbalances, such as hypokalemia, hyperkalemia, hypomagnesemia, and hypocalcemia
- metabolic acidosis
- hypoxia
- myocardial ischemia
- drug intoxication, particularly cocaine, amphetamines, and tricyclic antidepressants
- enlargement of the ventricular chambers
- increased sympathetic stimulation
- myocarditis.

This could get serious

PVCs are significant for two reasons. First, they can lead to more serious arrhythmias, such as ventricular tachycardia or ventricular fibrillation. The risk of developing a more serious arrhythmia increases in patients with ischemic or damaged hearts.

PVCs also decrease cardiac output, especially if the ectopic beats are frequent or sustained. Decreased cardiac output is caused by reduced ventricular diastolic filling time and a loss of atrial kick. The clinical impact of PVCs hinges on how well perfusion is maintained and how long the abnormal rhythm lasts.

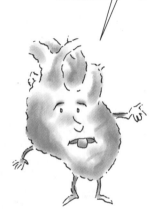

The risk is greater in people with damaged hearts.

Don't skip this strip

Identifying PVCs

This ECG strip shows premature ventricular contractions (PVCs) on beats 1, 6, and 11. Note the wide and bizarre appearance of the QRS complex.

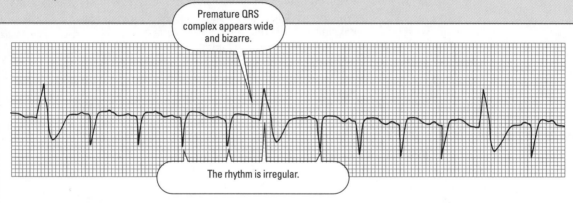

Premature QRS complex appears wide and bizarre.

The rhythm is irregular.

- *Rhythm:* irregular
- *Rate:* 120 beats/minute
- *P wave:* none with PVC, but P wave present with other QRS complexes

- *PR interval:* 0.12 second in underlying rhythm
- *QRS complex:* early, with bizarre configuration and duration of 0.14 second in PVC; QRS complexes are 0.08 second in underlying rhythm

- *T wave:* normal; opposite direction from QRS complex
- *QT interval:* 0.28 second with underlying rhythm
- *Other:* none

What to look for

On the ECG strip, PVCs look wide and bizarre and appear as early beats causing atrial and ventricular irregularity. The rate follows the underlying rhythm, which is usually regular.

The P wave is usually absent. Retrograde P waves may be stimulated by the PVC and cause distortion of the ST segment. The PR interval and QT interval aren't measurable on a premature beat, only on the normal beats.

Complex configuration

The QRS complex occurs early. Configuration of the QRS complex is usually normal in the underlying rhythm. The duration of the QRS complex in the premature beat exceeds 0.12 second. The

T wave in the premature beat has a deflection opposite that of the QRS complex.

When a PVC strikes on the downslope of the preceding normal T wave—the R-on-T phenomenon—it can trigger more serious rhythm disturbances.

The pause that compensates

A horizontal baseline called a compensatory pause may follow the T wave of the PVC. When a compensatory pause appears, the interval between two normal sinus beats containing a PVC equals two normal sinus intervals. (See *Compensatory pause.*) This pause occurs because the ventricle is refractory and can't respond to the next regularly timed P wave from the sinus node. When a compensatory pause doesn't occur, the PVC is referred to as interpolated.

PVCs all in a row

PVCs that look alike are called unifocal and originate from the same ectopic focus. These beats may also appear in patterns that can progress to more lethal arrhythmias. (See *When PVCs spell danger.*)

Ruling out trouble

To help determine the seriousness of PVCs, ask yourself these questions:

• How often do they occur? In patients with chronic PVCs, an increase in frequency or a change in the pattern of PVCs from the baseline rhythm may signal a more serious condition.

• What pattern do they occur in? If the ECG shows a dangerous pattern—such as paired PVCs, PVCs with more than one focus, bigeminy, or R-on-T phenomenon—the patient may require immediate treatment.

• Are they really PVCs? Make sure the complex you see is a PVC, not another, less dangerous arrhythmia. (See *Deciphering PVCs.*) Don't delay treatment, however, if the patient is unstable.

Outward signs tell a story

The patient with PVCs will have a much weaker pulse wave after the premature beat and a longer-than-normal pause between pulse waves. At times, you won't be able to palpate any pulse after the PVC. If the carotid pulse is visible, however, you may see a weaker pulse wave after the premature beat. When auscultating for heart sounds, you'll hear an abnormally early heart sound and a diminished amplitude with each premature beat.

Patients with frequent PVCs may complain of palpitations and may also experience hypotension or syncope.

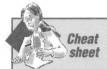

Cheat sheet

Recognizing a PVC

• *Rhythm:* irregular during PVC; underlying rhythm may be regular
• *Rate:* follows underlying rhythm
• *P wave:* absent
• *PR interval:* unmeasurable
• *QRS complex:* wide and bizarre
• *T wave:* opposite direction from QRS complex
• *QT interval:* unmeasurable
• *Other:* possible compensatory pause

Compensatory pause

You can determine if a compensatory pause exists by using calipers to mark off two normal P-P intervals. Place one leg of the calipers on the sinus P wave that comes just before the PVC. If the pause is compensatory, the other leg of the calipers will fall precisely on the P wave that comes after the pause.

When PVCs spell danger

Here are some examples of patterns of dangerous premature ventricular contractions (PVCs).

Paired PVCs

Two PVCs in a row are called a pair or couplet (see highlighted areas). A pair can produce ventricular tachycardia because the second contraction usually meets refractory tissue. A salvo—three or more PVCs in a row—is considered a run of ventricular tachycardia.

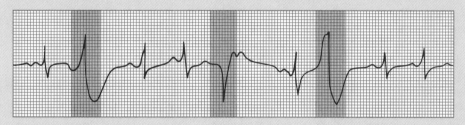

Multiform PVCs

PVCs that look different from one another arise from different sites or from the same site with abnormal conduction (see highlighted areas). Multiform PVCs may indicate severe heart disease or digoxin toxicity.

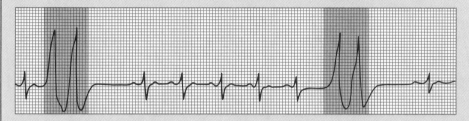

Bigeminy and trigeminy

PVCs that occur every other beat (bigeminy) or every third beat (trigeminy) can result in ventricular tachycardia or ventricular fibrillation (see highlighted areas).

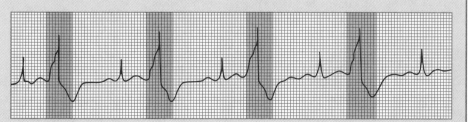

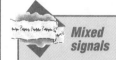

Mixed signals

Deciphering PVCs

To determine whether the rhythm you're assessing is a premature ventricular contraction (PVC) or some other beat, ask yourself the following questions:
• Are you seeing ventricular escape beats rather than PVCs? Escape beats act as a safety mechanism to protect the heart from ventricular standstill.
• Are you seeing normal beats with aberrant ventricular conduction? Some supraventricular impulses may take an abnormal pathway through the ventricular conduction system, causing the QRS complex to appear abnormal.

(continued)

When PVCs spell danger (continued)

R-on-T phenomenon

In R-on-T phenomenon, the PVC occurs so early that it falls on the T wave of the preceding beat (see highlighted area). Because the cells haven't fully repolarized, ventricular tachycardia or ventricular fibrillation can result.

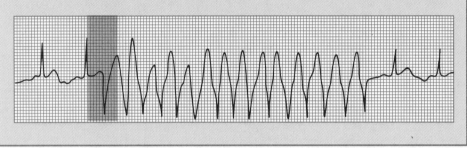

Cheat sheet

Signs of PVC

- Much weaker pulse wave after the premature beat
- Longer-than-normal pause between pulse waves
- When auscultating for heart sounds, abnormally early heart sound and diminished amplitude with each premature beat

How you intervene

If the patient is asymptomatic and doesn't have heart disease, the arrhythmia probably won't require treatment. If he has symptoms or a dangerous form of PVCs, the type of treatment depends on the cause of the problem.

If the PVCs have a cardiac origin, the doctor may order drugs to suppress ventricular irritability such as procainamide or lidocaine. Procainamide may be given in an infusion at a maintenance dose of 1 to 4 mg/minute. After an I.V. bolus of 1 to 1.5 mg/kg of lidocaine, you may give an infusion of 1 to 4 mg/minute.

When PVCs have a noncardiac origin, treatment is aimed at correcting the cause. This could mean, for example, adjusting drug therapy or correcting acidosis, electrolyte imbalances, hypothermia, or hypoxia.

Stat assessment

Patients who have recently developed PVCs need prompt assessment, especially if they have underlying heart disease or complex medical problems. Those with chronic PVCs should be observed closely for the development of more frequent PVCs or more dangerous PVC patterns. (See *Key facts about PVCs*.)

Until effective treatment is begun, patients with PVCs accompanied by serious symptoms should have continuous ECG monitoring and ambulate only with assistance. If the patient is discharged from the hospital on antiarrhythmic medications, family members should know how to contact the emergency medical

Key facts about PVCs

- PVCs may be benign or a warning sign of impending lethal arrhythmias.
- The QRS complex is wide and bizarre.
- PVCs have a variety of patterns.
- Treatment for PVCs varies with the cause and the patient's symptoms.

system and how to perform cardiopulmonary resuscitation (CPR).

Idioventricular rhythms

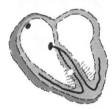

Called the rhythms of last resort, idioventricular rhythms act as safety mechanisms to prevent ventricular standstill when no impulses are conducted to the ventricles from above the bundle of His. The cells of the His-Purkinje system take over and act as the heart's pacemaker to generate electrical impulses.

Idioventricular rhythms can occur as ventricular escape beats, idioventricular rhythm (a term used to designate a specific type of idioventricular rhythm), or accelerated idioventricular rhythm. (See *Key facts about idioventricular rhythm.*)

How it happens

Idioventricular rhythms occur when all of the heart's other pacemakers fail to function or when supraventricular impulses can't reach the ventricles because of a block in the conduction system. The arrhythmias may accompany third-degree heart block or be caused by:
• myocardial ischemia
• myocardial infarction (MI)
• digoxin toxicity
• pacemaker failure
• metabolic imbalances.

Conduction foibles and pacemaker failures

Idioventricular rhythms signal a serious conduction defect with a failure of the primary pacemaker. The slow ventricular rate of these arrhythmias and the loss of atrial kick markedly reduce cardiac output. Patients bear close watching because this problem can progress to more lethal arrhythmias. Idioventricular arrhythmias also commonly occur in dying patients.

What to look for

If just one idioventricular beat is generated, it's called a ventricular escape beat. (See *Identifying idioventricular rhythm,* page 130.) The beat appears late in the conduction cycle, when the rate drops to 40 beats/minute.

Consecutive ventricular beats on the ECG strip make up idioventricular rhythm. When this arrhythmia occurs, atrial rhythm

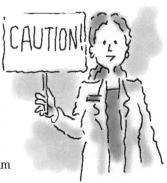

> ### Key facts about idioventricular rhythm
>
> • Higher pacemakers fail to conduct impulses to the ventricles, so the ventricles take over.
> • The idioventricular rate is generally 20 to 40 beats/minute, though it can be as high as 40 to 100 beats/minute (accelerated idioventricular rhythm).
> • QRS complexes are wide and bizarre.
> • Patients require treatment because they may become unstable with markedly reduced cardiac output.

and rate can't be determined. The ventricular rhythm is usually regular at 20 to 40 beats/minute, the inherent rate of the ventricles. If the rate is faster, it's called an accelerated idioventricular rhythm. (*See Accelerated idioventricular rhythm.*)

A telltale arrhythmia

Distinguishing characteristics of idioventricular rhythm include an absent P wave or one that can't conduct through to the ventricles. This makes the PR interval unmeasurable.

Because of abnormal ventricular depolarization, the QRS complex has a duration of longer than 0.12 second, with a wide and bizarre configuration. The T-wave deflection may be opposite the QRS complex. The QT interval is usually prolonged, indicating delayed depolarization and repolarization.

The patient may complain of palpitations, dizziness, or lightheadedness, or he may have a syncopal episode. If the arrhythmia

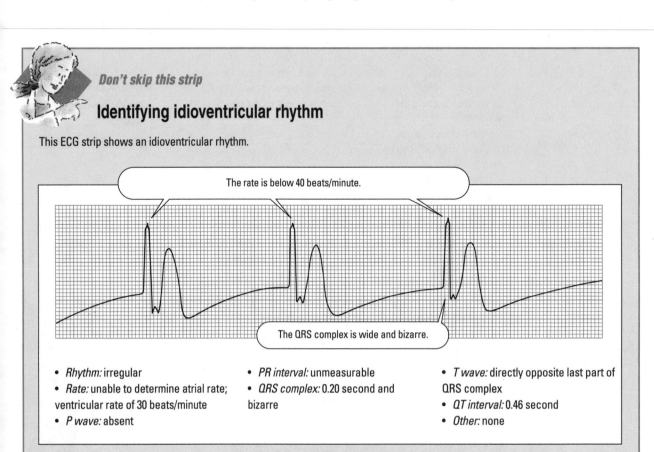

Don't skip this strip

Identifying idioventricular rhythm

This ECG strip shows an idioventricular rhythm.

The rate is below 40 beats/minute.

The QRS complex is wide and bizarre.

- *Rhythm:* irregular
- *Rate:* unable to determine atrial rate; ventricular rate of 30 beats/minute
- *P wave:* absent

- *PR interval:* unmeasurable
- *QRS complex:* 0.20 second and bizarre

- *T wave:* directly opposite last part of QRS complex
- *QT interval:* 0.46 second
- *Other:* none

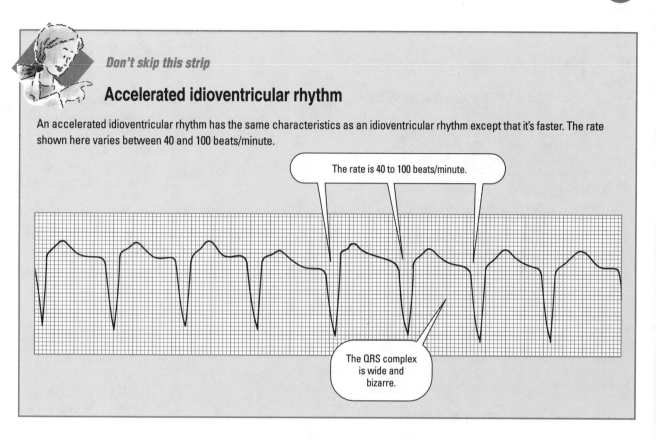

Don't skip this strip

Accelerated idioventricular rhythm

An accelerated idioventricular rhythm has the same characteristics as an idioventricular rhythm except that it's faster. The rate shown here varies between 40 and 100 beats/minute.

The rate is 40 to 100 beats/minute.

The QRS complex is wide and bizarre.

persists, hypotension, weak peripheral pulses, decreased urine output, or confusion can occur.

How you intervene

Treatment should be initiated immediately to increase the patient's heart rate, improve cardiac output, and establish a normal rhythm. Atropine may be prescribed to increase the heart rate.

If atropine isn't effective or if the patient develops hypotension or other signs of instability, a pacemaker may be needed to reestablish a heart rate that provides enough cardiac output to perfuse organs properly. A transcutaneous pacemaker may be used in an emergency until a temporary or permanent transvenous pacemaker can be inserted. (See *Transcutaneous pacemaker*, page 132.)

Remember that the goal of treatment doesn't include suppressing the idioventricular rhythm because it acts as a safety mechanism to protect the heart from standstill. *Idioventricular rhythm*

I can't waste time

Transcutaneous pacemaker

In life-threatening situations in which time is critical, a transcutaneous pacemaker may be used to regulate the heart rate. This device sends an electrical impulse from the pulse generator to the heart by way of two electrodes placed on the patient's chest and back, as shown.

The electrodes are placed at heart level, on either side of the heart, so the electrical stimulus has only a short distance to travel to the heart. Transcutaneous pacing is quick and effective, but it's used only until transvenous pacing can be started.

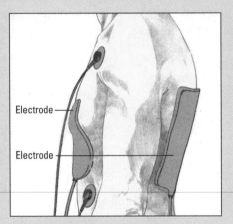

Electrode

Electrode

Cheat sheet

Recognizing idioventricular rhythm

- *Rhythm:* atrial undetermined; ventricular usually regular
- *Rate:* atrial unmeasurable; ventricular 20 to 40 beats/minute
- *P wave:* absent
- *PR interval:* unmeasurable
- *QRS complex:* wide and bizarre
- *T wave:* deflection opposite that of QRS complex
- *QT interval:* greater than 0.44 second
- *Other:* none

should never be treated with lidocaine or other antiarrhythmics that would suppress that safety mechanism.

Continuous monitoring needed

Patients with idioventricular rhythms need continuous ECG monitoring and constant assessment until treatment restores hemodynamic stability. Keep atropine and pacemaker equipment at the bedside. Enforce bed rest until a permanent system is in place for maintaining an effective heart rate.

Be sure to tell the patient and family members about the serious nature of this arrhythmia and all aspects of treatment. If a permanent pacemaker is inserted, teach the patient and family how it works, how to recognize problems, when to contact the doctor, and how pacemaker function will be monitored.

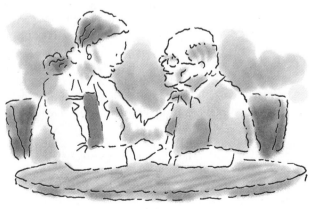

Ventricular tachycardia

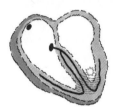

In ventricular tachycardia, commonly called V-tach, three or more PVCs occur in a row and the ventricular rate exceeds 100 beats/minute. This arrhythmia usually precedes ventricular fibrillation and sudden cardiac death, especially in patients who aren't in the hospital.

Ventricular tachycardia is an extremely unstable rhythm. It can occur in short, paroxysmal bursts lasting fewer than 30 seconds and causing few or no symptoms. Alternatively, it can be sustained, requiring immediate treatment to prevent death, even in patients initially able to maintain adequate cardiac output. (See *Key facts about V-tach.*)

How it happens

This arrhythmia usually results from increased myocardial irritability, which may be triggered by enhanced automaticity or reentry within the Purkinje system or by PVCs initiating the R-on-T phenomenon. Conditions that can cause ventricular tachycardia include:
- myocardial ischemia
- MI
- coronary artery disease
- valvular heart disease
- heart failure
- cardiomyopathy
- electrolyte imbalances such as hypokalemia
- drug intoxication from digoxin, procainamide, quinidine, or cocaine.

Unpredictable V-tach

Ventricular tachycardia is significant because of its unpredictability and potential to cause death. A patient may be stable with a normal pulse and adequate hemodynamics or unstable with hypotension and no detectable pulse. Because of reduced ventricular filling time and the drop in cardiac output, the patient's condition can quickly deteriorate to ventricular fibrillation and complete cardiac collapse.

What to look for

On the ECG strip, the atrial rhythm and rate can't be determined. The ventricular rhythm is usually regular but may be slightly irreg-

> ## Key facts about V-tach
>
> - Ventricular tachycardia (V-tach) occurs when three or more premature ventricular contractions occur in a row.
> - The rate is 100 to 200 beats/minute.
> - The condition of the patient with this arrhythmia may or may not be stable. The rhythm can severely compromise cardiac output and create an emergency situation.
> - Treatment varies with the patient's condition. He may be pulseless and require cardiopulmonary resuscitation, or he may have a pulse and need medications or cardioversion.

ular. The ventricular rate is usually rapid — 100 to 200 beats/minute.

The P wave is usually absent but may be obscured by the QRS complex. Retrograde P waves may be present. Because the P wave can't be seen in most cases, you can't measure the PR interval. The QRS complex has a bizarre configuration, usually with an increased amplitude and a duration of longer than 0.14 second.

All about uniformity

QRS complexes in monomorphic ventricular tachycardia have a uniform shape. In polymorphic ventricular tachycardia, the shape of the QRS complex constantly changes. If the T wave is visible, it occurs opposite the QRS complex. The QT interval isn't measurable. (See *Identifying ventricular tachycardia.*)

Torsades de pointes is a special variation of polymorphic ventricular tachycardia. (See *Torsades de pointes.*)

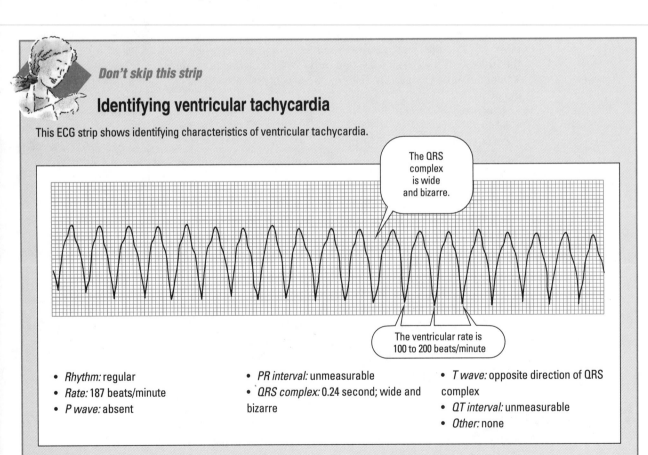

Don't skip this strip

Identifying ventricular tachycardia

This ECG strip shows identifying characteristics of ventricular tachycardia.

The QRS complex is wide and bizarre.

The ventricular rate is 100 to 200 beats/minute

- *Rhythm:* regular
- *Rate:* 187 beats/minute
- *P wave:* absent

- *PR interval:* unmeasurable
- *QRS complex:* 0.24 second; wide and bizarre

- *T wave:* opposite direction of QRS complex
- *QT interval:* unmeasurable
- *Other:* none

Don't skip this strip

Torsades de pointes

Torsades de pointes, which means "twisting about the points," is a special form of polymorphic ventricular tachycardia. The hallmark characteristics of this rhythm, shown below, are QRS complexes that rotate about the baseline, deflecting downward and upward for several beats.

The rate is 150 to 250 beats/minute, usually with an irregular rhythm, and the QRS complexes are wide. The P wave is usually absent.

Paroxysmal rhythm
This arrhythmia may be paroxysmal, starting and stopping suddenly, and may deteriorate into ventricular fibrillation. It should be considered when ventricular tachycardia doesn't respond to antiarrhythmic therapy or other treatments.

Reversible causes
The cause of this form of ventricular tachycardia is usually reversible. The most common causes are drugs that lengthen the QT interval, such as the antiarrhythmics quinidine, procainamide, and sotalol. Other causes include myocardial ischemia and electrolyte abnormalities, such as hypokalemia, hypomagnesemia, and hypocalcemia.

Going into overdrive
Torsades de pointes is treated by correcting the underlying cause, especially if the cause is related to specific drug therapy. The doctor may order mechanical overdrive pacing, which overrides the ventricular rate and breaks the triggered mechanism for the arrhythmia. Magnesium sulfate may also be effective. Electrical cardioversion may be used when torsades de pointes doesn't respond to other treatment.

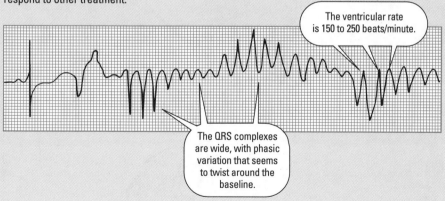

The ventricular rate is 150 to 250 beats/minute.

The QRS complexes are wide, with phasic variation that seems to twist around the baseline.

Quick work prevents collapse

Although some patients have only minor symptoms at first, they still need rapid intervention and treatment to prevent cardiac collapse. Most patients with ventricular tachycardia have weak or absent pulses. Low cardiac output will cause hypotension and a decreased level of consciousness leading to unresponsiveness. Ventricular tachycardia may precipitate angina, heart failure, or a substantial decrease in organ perfusion.

How you intervene

Treatment depends on whether the patient's pulse is detectable or undetectable. Patients with pulseless ventricular tachycardia receive the same treatment as those with ventricular fibrillation and require immediate resuscitation. Treatment for patients with a detectable pulse depends on whether their condition is stable or unstable.

Unstable patients generally have heart rates greater than 150 beats/minute. They may also have hypotension, shortness of breath, an altered level of consciousness, heart failure, angina, or MI—conditions that indicate cardiac decompensation. These patients are treated immediately with direct-current synchronized cardioversion.

Understanding the implantable cardioverter-defibrillator

The implantable cardioverter-defibrillator (ICD) has a programmable pulse generator and lead system that monitors the heart's activity, detects ventricular arrhythmias and tachyarrhythmias, and responds with appropriate therapies. The range of therapies includes antitachycardia and antibradycardia pacing, cardioversion, and defibrillation. Newer defibrillators also have the ability to pace both the atrium and ventricle.

Implantation of the ICD is similar to that of a permanent pacemaker. The cardiologist positions the lead (or leads) transvenously in the endocardium of the right ventricle (and the right atrium, if both chambers require pacing). The lead connects to a generator box, which is implanted in the right or left upper chest near the clavicle.

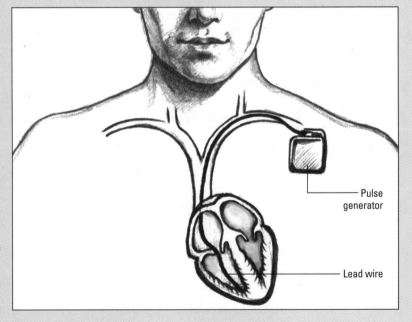

Pulse generator

Lead wire

Typical tachycardia complex

A stable patient with a wide QRS complex tachycardia and no signs of cardiac decompensation is treated differently. First, if the patient has monomorphic ventricular tachycardia, procainamide is given to try to correct the rhythm disturbance; then other drugs such as amiodarone are used. If the patient becomes unstable, immediate synchronized cardioversion is performed. If the patient has polymorphic ventricular tachycardia, a beta-adrenergic blocker, amiodarone, or procainamide may be given.

Patients with chronic, recurrent episodes of ventricular tachycardia who are unresponsive to drug therapy may have a cardioverter-defibrillator implanted. This device is a more permanent solution to recurrent episodes of ventricular tachycardia. (See *Understanding the implantable cardioverter-defibrillator.*)

Always assume the worst

Any wide QRS complex tachycardia should be treated as ventricular tachycardia until definitive evidence is found to establish another diagnosis, such as supraventricular tachycardia with abnormal ventricular conduction. *Always assume that the patient has ventricular tachycardia and treat him accordingly. Rapid intervention will prevent cardiac decompensation or the onset of more lethal arrhythmias.*

Teacher, teacher

Be sure to teach patients and families about the serious nature of this arrhythmia and the need for prompt treatment. If your patient is undergoing cardioversion, tell him he'll be given an analgesic or a sedative to help prevent discomfort.

If a patient will be discharged with an implanted defibrillator or a prescription for long-term antiarrhythmic medications, teach his family how to contact the emergency medical system and how to perform CPR.

Ventricular fibrillation

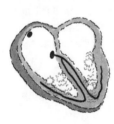

Ventricular fibrillation, commonly called V-fib, is a chaotic pattern of electrical activity in the ventricles in which electrical impulses arise from many different foci. It produces no effective muscular contraction and no cardiac output. Untreated ventricular fibrillation causes most cases of sudden cardiac death in people outside of a hospital.

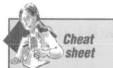

Cheat sheet

Recognizing ventricular tachycardia

• *Rhythm:* atrial rhythm can't be determined; regular or slightly irregular ventricular rhythm
• *Rate:* atrial rate can't be determined; ventricular rate of 100 to 200 beats/minute
• *P wave:* absent or obscured by QRS complex
• *PR interval:* unmeasurable
• *QRS complex:* wide and bizarre; duration longer than 0.12 second
• *T wave:* opposite direction of QRS complex
• *QT interval:* unmeasurable
• *Other:* torsades de pointes may be seen.

How it happens

Causes of ventricular fibrillation include:
- myocardial ischemia
- MI
- untreated ventricular tachycardia
- underlying heart disease
- acid-base imbalance
- electric shock
- severe hypothermia
- electrolyte imbalances, such as hypokalemia, hyperkalemia, and hypercalcemia.

Quivering ventricles

With ventricular fibrillation, the ventricles quiver instead of contract, so cardiac output falls to zero. If fibrillation continues, it leads to ventricular standstill and death.

What to look for

On the ECG strip, ventricular activity appears as fibrillatory waves with no recognizable pattern. Atrial rate and rhythm can't be determined, nor can ventricular rhythm because no pattern or regularity occurs.

As a result, the ventricular rate, P wave, PR interval, QRS complex, T wave, and QT interval can't be determined. Larger, or coarse, fibrillatory waves are easier to convert to a normal rhythm than are smaller waves because larger waves indicate a greater degree of electrical activity in the heart. (See *Identifying ventricular fibrillation.*)

No greater urgency

The patient in ventricular fibrillation is in full cardiac arrest, unresponsive, and without a detectable blood pressure or carotid or femoral pulse. Whenever you see a pattern resembling ventricular fibrillation, check the rhythm in another lead, check the patient immediately, and start treatment. (See *Treating ventricular fibrillation.*)

Be aware that other things can mimic ventricular fibrillation on an ECG strip. Interference from an electric razor is one such mimic, as is muscle movement from shivering.

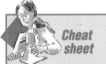

Recognizing ventricular fibrillation

- *Rhythm:* can't be determined
- *Rate:* can't be determined
- *P wave:* can't be determined
- *PR interval:* can't be determined
- *QRS complex:* can't be determined
- *T wave:* can't be determined
- *QT interval:* not applicable
- *Other:* variable size of fibrillatory waves

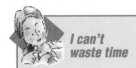

I can't waste time

Treating ventricular fibrillation

- Check the rhythm strip in another lead.
- Check the patient immediately.
- Start treatment—CPR followed by immediate defibrillation.

Don't skip this strip

Identifying ventricular fibrillation

The first ECG strip shows coarse ventricular fibrillation; the second shows fine ventricular fibrillation.

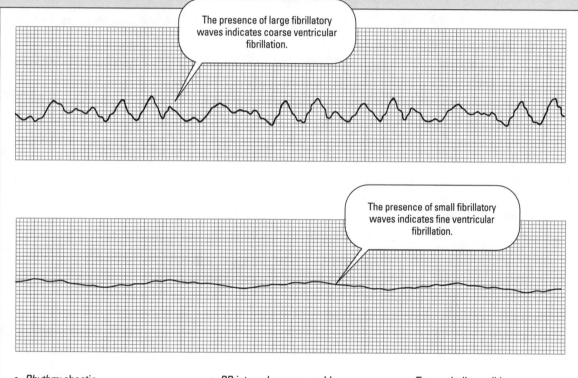

The presence of large fibrillatory waves indicates coarse ventricular fibrillation.

The presence of small fibrillatory waves indicates fine ventricular fibrillation.

- *Rhythm:* chaotic
- *Rate:* undetermined
- *P wave:* absent
- *PR interval:* unmeasurable
- *QRS complex:* indiscernible
- *T wave:* indiscernible
- *QT interval:* not applicable
- *Other:* waveform is a wavy line

How you intervene

Defibrillation is the most effective treatment for ventricular fibrillation. (See *Treating ventricular fibrillation or pulseless ventricular tachycardia*, pages 140 and 141.) CPR must be performed until the defibrillator arrives to preserve oxygen supply to the brain

(Text continues on page 142.)

Treating ventricular fibrillation or pulseless ventricular tachycardia

The following algorithm, based on the most recent information from the American Heart Association, shows the critical steps to take during cardiac arrest caused by ventricular fibrillation (VF) or pulseless ventricular tachycardia (VT).

- Assess airway, breathing, and circulation.
- Perform cardiopulmonary resuscitation (CPR) until the defibrillator is attached.
- Administer precordial thump *if you witnessed the arrest and the patient has no pulse and if a defibrillator isn't immediately available.*
- Confirm VF or pulseless VT on the defibrillator, and confirm the absence of a pulse.

Defibrillate as many as three times (200 to 300 joules, then 360 joules) as needed for persistent VF or pulseless VT.

Determine the heart rhythm.

Pulseless electrical activity is present.

Spontaneous circulation returns.
- Assess vital signs.
- Support airway.
- Support breathing.
- Provide medications appropriate for maintaining blood pressure and heart rate and rhythm.

- Continue CPR.
- Intubate at once.
- Establish an I.V. line
- Assess blood flow using Doppler ultrasound.

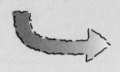

Consider possible causes and anticipate treatment. Causes include:
- hypovolemia
- hypoxia
- cardiac tamponade
- tension pneumothorax
- hypothermia
- massive pulmonary embolism
- overdose of drugs, for example, tricyclic antidepressants, digoxin, beta-adrenergic blockers, or calcium channel blockers
- hyperkalemia
- massive acute myocardial infarction.

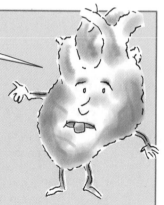

Defibrillation is the key to getting me back on the right track.

Asystole is present. Refer to the algorithm on page 145.

Persistent or recurring VF or pulseless VT is present.
• Continue CPR.
• Intubate at once.
• Establish an I.V. line.
• Administer epinephrine, 1 mg I.V. push. Repeat every 3 to 5 minutes.
Or administer vasopressin 40 U I.V. as a single one-time dose. (if no response after single dose of vasopressin, may give epinephrine 1 mg I.V. every 3 to 5 minutes).

Defibrillate with 360 joules within 30 to 60 seconds.

Administer prescribed medications, which may include one or more of the following:
• amiodarone 300 mg I.V. push. If VF/pulseless VT recurs, consider second dose of 150 mg I.V. Maximum dose 2.2 g over 24 hours.
• lidocaine, 1 to 1.5 mg/kg I.V. push. Repeat every 3 to 5 minutes to a maximum of 3 mg/kg.
• magnesium sulfate, 1 to 2 g I.V. in torsades de pointes.
• procainamide, 30 mg/minute to a maximum of 17 mg/kg.

Administer epinephrine, 1 mg I.V. push. Repeat every 3 to 5 minutes as needed.

For absolute bradycardia (below 60 beats/minute) or relative bradycardia, administer atropine, 1 mg I.V. Repeat every 3 to 5 minutes to a maximum of 0.04 mg/kg.

Defibrillate with 360 joules 30 to 60 seconds after each dose of medication or each minute of CPR. (The pattern should be *drug, shock, drug, shock.*)

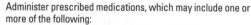

and other vital organs. Drugs such as epinephrine or vasopressin may help the heart respond better to defibrillation. Amiodarone and magnesium may be given to decrease heart irritability and prevent a recurrence of ventricular fibrillation.

A shock for life

During defibrillation, electrode paddles direct an electrical current through the patient's heart. The current causes the myocardium to depolarize, which, in turn, encourages the sinoatrial node to resume normal control of the heart's electrical activity.

One paddle is placed to the right of the upper sternum, and one is placed over the fifth or sixth intercostal space at the left anterior axillary line. During cardiac surgery, internal paddles are placed directly on the myocardium.

Automated-external defibrillators are increasingly being used to provide early defibrillation. In this method, electrode pads are placed on the patient's chest and a microcomputer in the unit interprets the cardiac rhythm, providing the caregiver with step-by-step instructions on how to proceed. These defibrillators can be used by people without medical experience.

Speed is the key

For the patient with ventricular fibrillation, successful resuscitation requires rapid recognition of the problem and prompt defibrillation. (See *Key facts about V-fib.*) Many health care facilities and emergency medical systems have established protocols to help health care workers initiate prompt treatment. Be sure you know where your facility keeps its emergency equipment and how to recognize and deal with lethal arrhythmias.

You'll also need to teach your patient and his family how to contact the emergency medical system. Family members need instruction in CPR. Teach them about long-term therapies that prevent recurrent episodes of ventricular fibrillation, including chronic antiarrhythmic drugs and implantation of a cardioverter-defibrillator.

> ### Key facts about V-fib
>
> • Ventricular fibrillation (V-fib) is an emergency because cardiac output is absent.
> • The fibrillatory pattern may be coarse or fine.
> • Immediate cardiopulmonary resuscitation and defibrillation are necessary for the patient's survival.

Asystole

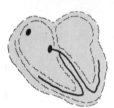

Asystole is ventricular standstill. The patient is completely unresponsive, with no electrical activity in the heart and no cardiac output. This arrhythmia results most often from a prolonged period of cardiac arrest without effective resuscitation.

Asystole has been called the arrhythmia of death. The patient is in cardiopulmonary arrest. Without rapid initiation of CPR and appropriate treatment, the situation quickly becomes irreversible.

How it happens

Anything that causes inadequate blood flow to the heart may lead to asystole, including:

- MI
- severe electrolyte disturbances such as hyperkalemia
- massive pulmonary embolism
- prolonged hypoxemia
- severe, uncorrected acid-base disturbances
- electric shock
- drug intoxication, such as cocaine overdose.

What to look for

On the ECG strip, asystole looks like a nearly flat line (except for changes caused by chest compressions during CPR). (See *Key facts about asystole.*) No electrical activity is evident, except possibly P waves for a time. Atrial and ventricular activity is at a standstill, so no intervals can be measured. (See *Identifying asystole.*)

In the patient with a pacemaker, pacer spikes may be evident on the strip, but no P wave or QRS complex occurs in response to the stimulus.

Key facts about asystole

- Ventricular activity is absent, and the patient has no cardiac output.
- Asystole appears as a nearly flat line on the ECG strip.
- This is a medical emergency. Start cardiopulmonary resuscitation and other resuscitation measures immediately.

Don't skip this strip

Identifying asystole

This ECG strip shows asystole, the absence of electrical activity in the ventricles. Except for a few P waves or pacer spikes, nothing appears on the waveform and the line is almost flat.

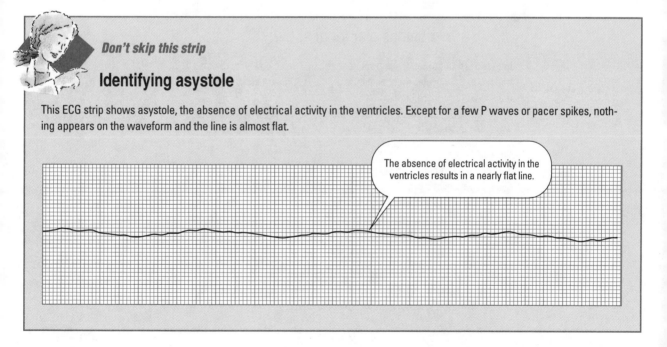

The absence of electrical activity in the ventricles results in a nearly flat line.

The patient will be unresponsive, without any discernible pulse or blood pressure.

How you intervene

The immediate treatment for asystole is CPR. (See *Treating asystole*.) Start CPR as soon as you determine that the patient has no pulse. Then verify the presence of asystole by checking two different ECG leads. Give repeated doses of epinephrine, as ordered.

Subsequent treatment for asystole focuses on identifying and either treating or removing the underlying cause. Transcutaneous pacing may also be considered.

Slim hope

Your job is to recognize this life-threatening arrhythmia and start resuscitation right away. Unfortunately, most patients with asystole can't be resuscitated, especially after a prolonged period of cardiac arrest.

You should also be aware that pulseless electrical activity can lead to asystole. Know how to recognize this problem and treat it. (See *Pulseless electrical activity*.)

I can't waste time

Pulseless electrical activity

In pulseless electrical activity, the heart muscle loses its ability to contract even though electrical activity is preserved. As a result, the patient goes into cardiac arrest.

On an ECG, you'll see evidence of organized electrical activity, but you won't be able to palpate a pulse or measure the blood pressure.

Causes
This condition requires rapid identification and treatment. Causes include hypovolemia, hypoxia, acidosis, tension pneumothorax, cardiac tamponade, massive pulmonary embolism, hypothermia, hyperkalemia, massive acute myocardial infarction, and an overdose of drugs such as tricyclic antidepressants.

Treatment
CPR is the immediate treatment, along with epinephrine. Atropine may be given to patients with bradycardia. Subsequent treatment focuses on identifying and correcting the underlying cause.

Treating asystole

This algorithm for treating asystole is based on the most recent guidelines from the American Heart Association.

- Perform initial assessment.
- Assess airway, breathing, and circulation.
- Perform cardiopulmonary resuscitation.

- Intubate the patient at once.
- Establish an I.V. line.
- Confirm the diagnosis of asystole in more than one lead.

Consider possible causes, including:

- hypoxia
- hyperkalemia
- hypokalemia

- preexisting acidosis
- drug overdose
- hypothermia.

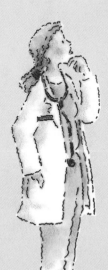

Consider performing transcutaneous pacing immediately.

Administer epinephrine, 1 mg I.V. push; repeat every 3 to 5 minutes.

Administer atropine, 1 mg I.V.; repeat every 3 to 5 minutes to a maximum of 0.04 mg/kg.

Consider terminating resuscitation efforts.

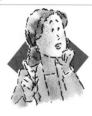

Quick quiz

1. PVCs are most dangerous if they:
   A.   are multiformed and increase in frequency.
   B.   appear wide and bizarre.
   C.   occur after the T wave.

Answer: A. PVCs that have different shapes and increase in frequency may signal severe heart disease or digoxin toxicity and progress to a lethal arrhythmia.

2. The treatment of choice for a patient with ventricular fibrillation is:
   A.   defibrillation.
   B.   transesophageal pacing.
   C.   synchronized cardioversion.

Answer: A. Patients with ventricular fibrillation are in cardiac arrest and require defibrillation.

3. Patients with a slow idioventricular rhythm that doesn't respond to atropine should receive:
   A.   lidocaine.
   B.   dobutamine.
   C.   transcutaneous pacing.

Answer: C. Transcutaneous pacing is a temporary way to increase the rate and ensure an adequate cardiac output. Neither lidocaine nor dobutamine are indicated for a slow idioventricular rhythm.

4. A compensatory pause occurs after a PVC because the:
   A.   atria conduct a retrograde impulse.
   B.   ventricle is refractory at that point.
   C.   bundle of His blocks sinus impulses to the ventricles.

Answer: B. A compensatory pause occurs because the ventricle is refractory and can't respond to the next regularly timed P wave from the sinus node.

5. The term pulseless electrical activity refers to a condition in which there is:
   A.   electrical activity in the heart but no actual contraction.
   B.   asystole on a monitor or rhythm strip.
   C.   an extremely slow heart rate but no pulse.

Answer: A. Pulseless electrical activity is electrical activity without mechanical contraction. The patient is in cardiac arrest, with no blood pressure or pulse.

Test strips

Ready to try a few test strips? Answer the questions below about each strip; then check your answers with ours.

6. In the strip below, the ventricular rhythm is irregular, the ventricular rate is 130 beats/minute, the P wave is absent, the PR interval and QT interval aren't measurable, the QRS complex is wide and bizarre with varying duration, and the T wave is opposite the QRS complex. You would interpret this rhythm as:
    A.   ventricular fibrillation.
    B.   ventricular tachycardia.
    C.   idioventricular rhythm.

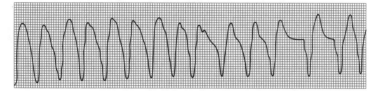

Answer: B. This strip shows ventricular tachycardia.

7. You would interpret the rhythm shown below as:
    A.   coarse ventricular fibrillation.
    B.   fine ventricular fibrillation.
    C.   torsades de pointes.

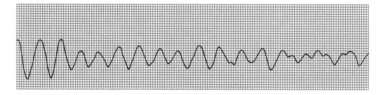

Answer: A. The ventricular rhythm is chaotic, the ventricular rate can't be determined, and the P wave, PR interval, QRS complex, T wave, and QT interval are indiscernible. These observations indicate coarse ventricular fibrillation.

Scoring

★★★ If you answered all seven questions correctly, sensational! You're
      simply the V-best!

★★   If you answered four to six questions correctly, super! You've got
     a great eye for V-rhythms!

★   If you answered fewer than four questions correctly, that's OK.
     Just monitor your V-heart away!

8

Atrioventricular blocks

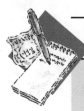

Just the facts

This chapter will show you how to identify atrioventricular (AV) block on an ECG and how the arrhythmias are treated. In this chapter, you'll learn:

♦ how to identify the various forms of AV block and interpret their rhythms

♦ why AV block is a significant arrhythmia

♦ which patients are at risk for developing AV block

♦ how to identify the signs and symptoms of AV block

♦ how to care for a patient with AV block.

A look at AV block

Atrioventricular (AV) heart block results from an interruption in the conduction of impulses between the atria and ventricles. AV block can be total or partial or it may delay conduction. The block can occur at the AV node, the bundle of His, or the bundle branches.

The heart's electrical impulses normally originate in the sinoatrial (SA) node, so when those impulses are blocked at the AV node, atrial rates are commonly normal (60 to 100 beats/minute). The clinical effect of the block depends on how many impulses are completely blocked, how slow the ventricular rate is as a result, and how the block ultimately affects the heart. A slow ventricular rate can decrease cardiac output, possibly causing lightheadedness, hypotension, and confusion.

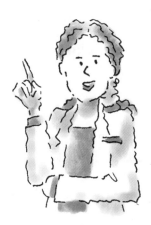

The cause before the block

A variety of factors may lead to AV block, including underlying heart conditions, use of certain drugs, congenital anomalies, and conditions that disrupt the cardiac conduction system. (See *Causes of AV block*, page 150.)

Typical examples include:

- myocardial ischemia, which impairs cellular function so cells repolarize more slowly or incompletely. The injured cells, in turn, may conduct impulses slowly or inconsistently. Relief of the ischemia can restore normal function to the AV node.
- myocardial infarction (MI), in which cell death occurs. If the necrotic cells are part of the conduction system, they no longer conduct impulses and a permanent AV block occurs.
- excessive dosage of or an exaggerated response to a drug, which can cause AV block or increase the likelihood that a block will develop. Although many antiarrhythmic medications can have this effect, the drugs more commonly known to cause or exacerbate AV blocks include digoxin, beta-adrenergic blockers, and calcium channel blockers.
- congenital anomalies such as congenital ventricular septal defect that involve cardiac structures and affect the conduction system. Anomalies of the conduction system, such as an AV node that doesn't conduct impulses, can also occur in the absence of structural defects.

Under the knife

AV block can also be caused by inadvertent damage to the heart's conduction system during cardiac surgery. Damage is most likely to occur in operations involving the mitral or tricuspid valve or in the closure of a ventricular septal defect. If the injury involves tissues adjacent to the surgical site and the conduction system isn't physically disrupted, the block may be only temporary. If a portion of the conduction system itself is severed, a permanent block results.

Radio blackout

Similar disruption of the conduction system can occur from a procedure called radiofrequency ablation. In this invasive procedure, a transvenous catheter is used to locate the area within the heart that participates in initiating or perpetuating certain tachyarrhythmias.

Radiofrequency energy is then delivered to the myocardium through this catheter to produce a small area of necrosis. The damaged tissue can no longer cause or participate in the tachyarrhythmia. If the energy is delivered close to the AV node, bundle of His, or bundle branches, block can occur.

Classes of block

AV blocks are classified according to their severity, not their location. That severity is measured according to how well the node

---

Causes of AV block

Atrioventricular (AV) blocks can be temporary or permanent. Here's a look at causes of each kind of AV block.

Causes of temporary block
- Myocardial infarction (MI), usually inferior wall
- Digoxin toxicity
- Acute myocarditis
- Calcium channel blockers
- Beta-adrenergic blockers
- Cardiac surgery

Causes of permanent block
- Changes associated with aging
- Congenital abnormalities
- MI, usually anteroseptal
- Cardiomyopathy
- Cardiac surgery

conducts impulses and is separated by degrees—first, second, and third. Let's take a look at them one at a time.

First-degree AV block

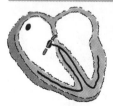

First-degree AV block occurs when impulses from the atria are consistently delayed during conduction through the AV node. Conduction eventually occurs; it just takes longer than normal. It's as if people are walking in a line through a doorway, but each person hesitates before crossing the threshold.

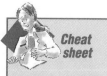

How it happens

First-degree AV block may appear normally in a healthy person or result from myocardial ischemia or infarction, myocarditis, or degenerative changes in the heart. The condition may also be caused by medications, such as digoxin, calcium channel blockers, and beta-adrenergic blockers.

First-degree AV block may be temporary, particularly if it stems from medications or ischemia early in the course of an MI. The presence of first-degree block, the least dangerous type of AV block, indicates some kind of problem in the conduction system. Because first-degree AV block can progress to a more severe block, it should be monitored for changes.

What to look for

In general, a rhythm strip with this block looks like normal sinus rhythm except that the PR interval is longer than normal. (See *Identifying first-degree AV block*, page 152.) The rhythm will be regular, with one normal P wave for every QRS complex.

The PR interval will be greater than 0.20 second and will be consistent for each beat. The QRS complex is usually normal, although sometimes a bundle-branch block may occur along with first-degree AV block and cause a widening of the QRS complex.

No signs of block

Most patients with first-degree AV block show no symptoms of the block because cardiac output isn't significantly affected. If the PR interval is extremely long, a longer interval between S_1 and S_2 may be noted on cardiac auscultation.

Cheat sheet

Signs of first-degree AV block

- *PR interval*—greater than 0.20 second; consistent for each beat
- No symptoms of block in most patients

Identifying first-degree AV block

The following rhythm strip shows first-degree AV block. Look for these distinguishing characteristics.

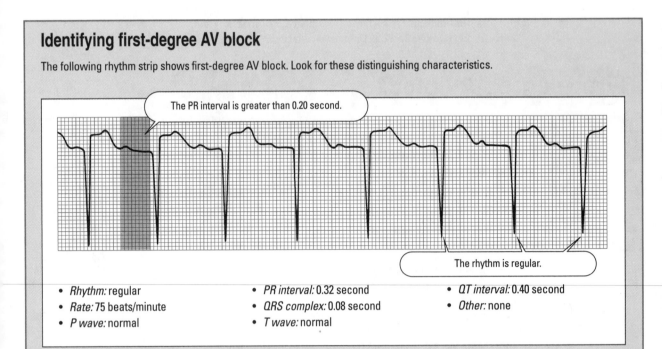

The PR interval is greater than 0.20 second.

The rhythm is regular.

- *Rhythm:* regular
- *Rate:* 75 beats/minute
- *P wave:* normal

- *PR interval:* 0.32 second
- *QRS complex:* 0.08 second
- *T wave:* normal

- *QT interval:* 0.40 second
- *Other:* none

How you intervene

Usually, just the underlying cause will be treated, not the conduction disturbance itself. For example, if a medication is causing the block, the dosage may be reduced or the medication may be discontinued. Close monitoring helps to detect progression of first-degree AV block to a more serious form of block.

When caring for a patient with first-degree AV block, evaluate him for underlying causes that can be corrected, such as medications or ischemia. Observe the electrocardiogram (ECG) for progression of the block to a more severe form of block. Administer digoxin, calcium channel blockers, or beta-adrenergic blockers cautiously.

Type I second-degree AV block

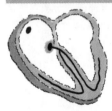

Also called Wenckebach or Mobitz type I block, type I second-degree AV block occurs when each successive impulse from the SA node is delayed slightly longer than the previous impulse. That pattern continues until an impulse fails to be conducted to the ventricles, and the cycle then repeats. It's like a line of people trying to get through a doorway, each one taking longer and longer until finally one can't get through.

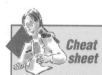

How it happens

Causes of type I second-degree AV block include coronary artery disease, inferior-wall MI, and rheumatic fever. It may also be due to cardiac medications, such as beta-adrenergic blockers, digoxin, and calcium channel blockers. Increased vagal stimulation can also cause this type of block.

Type I second-degree AV block may occur normally in an otherwise healthy person. Almost always temporary, this type of block resolves when the underlying condition is corrected. Although an asymptomatic patient with this block has a good prognosis, the block may progress to a more serious form, especially if it occurs early during an MI.

What to look for

When monitoring a patient with type I second-degree AV block, you'll note that because the SA node isn't affected by this lower block, it continues its normal activity. As a result, the atrial rhythm is normal. (See *Identifying type I second-degree AV block*, page 154.)

The PR interval gets gradually longer with each successive beat until finally a P wave fails to conduct to the ventricles. This makes the ventricular rhythm irregular, with a repeating pattern of groups of QRS complexes followed by a dropped beat in which the P wave isn't followed by a QRS complex.

Famous footprints

That pattern of grouped beating is sometimes referred to as the footprints of Wenckebach. (Karel Frederik Wenckebach was a Dutch internist who, at the turn of the century and long before the introduction of the ECG, described the two forms of what's now known as second-degree AV block by analyzing waves in the jugular venous pulse. Following the introduction of the ECG, German cardiologist Woldemar Mobitz clarified Wenckebach's findings as type I and type II).

When you're trying to identify type I second-degree AV block, think of the phrase "longer, longer, drop," which describes the progressively prolonged PR intervals and the missing QRS complex.

Cheat sheet

Signs of type I second-degree AV block

• *PR interval*—gradually gets longer with each beat until P wave fails to conduct to the ventricles
• *Ventricular rhythm*—irregular, with repeating pattern of groups of QRS complexes followed by a drop beat in which the P wave isn't followed by a QRS complex

Identifying type I second-degree AV block

The following rhythm strip illustrates type I second-degree AV block. Look for these distinguishing characteristics.

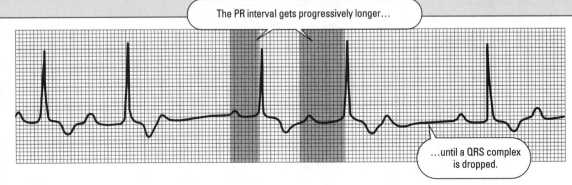

The PR interval gets progressively longer…

…until a QRS complex is dropped.

- *Rhythm:* atrial regular; ventricular irregular
- *Rate:* atrial 80 beats/minute; ventricular 50 beats/minute

- *P wave:* normal
- *PR interval:* progressively prolonged
- *QRS complex:* 0.08 second
- *T wave:* normal

- *QT interval:* 0.46 second
- *Other:* Wenckebach pattern of grouped beats

The QRS complexes, by the way, are usually normal because the delays occur in the AV node. (See *Rhythm strip patterns.*)

Lonely Ps, light-headed patients

Usually asymptomatic, a patient with type I second-degree AV block may show signs and symptoms of decreased cardiac output, such as light-headedness or hypotension. Symptoms may be especially pronounced if the ventricular rate is slow.

How you intervene

No treatment is needed if the patient is asymptomatic. For a symptomatic patient, atropine may improve AV node conduction. A temporary pacemaker may be required for long-term relief of symptoms until the rhythm resolves.

When caring for a patient with this block, assess his tolerance for the rhythm and the need for treatment to improve cardiac output. Evaluate the patient for possible causes of the block, including the use of certain medications or the presence of ischemia.

Check the ECG frequently to see if a more severe type of AV block develops. Make sure the patient has a patent I.V. line. Teach him about his temporary pacemaker, if indicated.

Rhythm strip patterns

The more you look at rhythm strips, the more you'll notice patterns. The symbols below represent some of the patterns you might see as you study rhythm strips.

Normal, regular (as in normal sinus rhythm)	♥	♥	♥	♥	♥	♥
Slow, regular (as in sinus bradycardia)	♥		♥			♥
Fast, regular (as in sinus tachycardia)	♥	♥	♥	♥	♥	♥
Premature (as in a premature ventricular contraction)	♥	♥	♥	♥	♥	♥
Grouped (as in type I second-degree AV block)	♥	♥	♥	♥	♥	♥
Irregularly irregular (as in atrial fibrillation)	♥	♥	♥	♥	♥	♥
Paroxysm or burst (as in paroxysmal atrial tachycardia)	♥	♥	♥	♥	♥	♥

Type II second-degree AV block

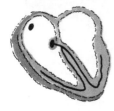

Type II second-degree AV block, also known as Mobitz type II block, is less common than type I but more serious. It occurs when occasional impulses from the SA node fail to conduct to the ventricles.

On an ECG, you won't see the PR interval lengthen before the impulse fails to conduct, as you do with type I second-degree AV block. You'll see, instead, consistent AV node conduction and an occasional dropped beat. This block is like a line of people passing through a doorway at the same speed, except that, periodically, one of them just can't get through.

How it happens

Type II second-degree AV block is usually caused by an anterior-wall MI, degenerative changes in the conduction system, or severe coronary artery disease. The arrhyth-

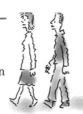
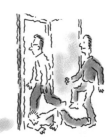

mia indicates a problem at the level of the bundle of His or bundle branches.

Type II block is more serious than type I because the ventricular rate tends to be slower and the cardiac output diminished. It's also more likely to cause symptoms, particularly if the sinus rhythm is slow and the ratio of conducted beats to dropped beats is low such as 2:1. Usually chronic, type II second-degree AV block may progress to a more serious form of block. (See *High-grade AV block.*)

Don't skip this strip

High-grade AV block

When two or more successive atrial impulses are blocked, the conduction disturbance is called high-grade atrioventricular (AV) block. Expressed as a ratio of atrial-to-ventricular beats, this block will be at least 3:1. With the prolonged refractory period of this block, latent pacemakers can discharge. As a result, you'll commonly see escape rhythms develop.

Complications

High-grade AV block causes severe complications. For instance, decreased cardiac output and reduced heart rate can combine to cause Stokes-Adams syncopal attacks. In addition, high-grade AV block often progresses quickly to third-degree block.

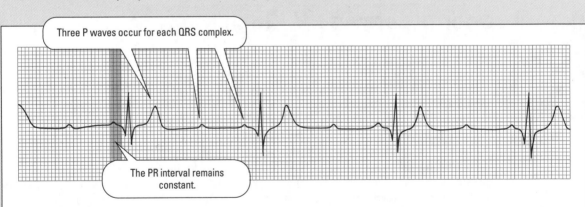

Three P waves occur for each QRS complex.

The PR interval remains constant.

- *Rhythm:* atrial usually regular; ventricular usually irregular
- *Rate:* atrial rate exceeds ventricular rate, usually below 40 beats/minute

- *P wave:* usually normal but some not followed by a QRS complex
- *PR interval:* constant but may be normal or prolonged

- *QRS complex:* usually normal, periodically absent
- *Other:* rhythm has appearance of complete AV block except for occasional conducted beat

Identifying type II second-degree AV block

The following rhythm strip shows type II second-degree atrioventricular (AV) block. Look for these distinguishing characteristics.

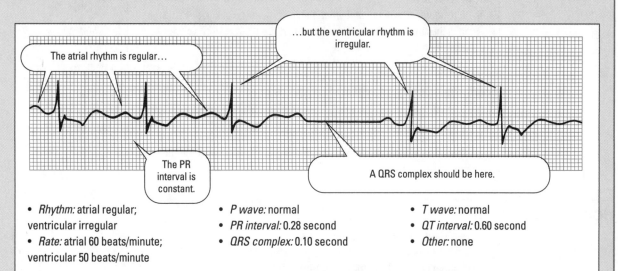

The atrial rhythm is regular…

…but the ventricular rhythm is irregular.

The PR interval is constant.

A QRS complex should be here.

- *Rhythm:* atrial regular; ventricular irregular
- *Rate:* atrial 60 beats/minute; ventricular 50 beats/minute

- *P wave:* normal
- *PR interval:* 0.28 second
- *QRS complex:* 0.10 second

- *T wave:* normal
- *QT interval:* 0.60 second
- *Other:* none

What to look for

When monitoring a rhythm strip, look for an atrial rhythm that's regular and a ventricular rhythm that may be regular or irregular, depending on the block. (See *Identifying type II second-degree AV block.*) If the block is intermittent, the rhythm is irregular. If the block is constant, such as 2:1 or 3:1, the rhythm is regular.

Overall, the strip will look as if someone erased some QRS complexes. The PR interval will be constant for all conducted beats but may be prolonged in some cases. The QRS complex is usually wide, but normal complexes may occur. (See *2:1 AV block,* page 158.)

Jumpin' palpitations!

Most patients who experience a few dropped beats remain asymptomatic as long as cardiac output is maintained. As the number of dropped beats increases, a patient may experience palpitations, fatigue, dyspnea, chest pain, or light-headedness. On physical ex-

2:1 AV block

In 2:1 second-degree atrioventricular (AV) block, every other QRS complex is dropped, so there are always two P waves for every QRS complex. The resulting ventricular rhythm is regular.

Type I or type II?

To help determine whether a rhythm is type I or type II block, look at the width of the QRS complexes. If they're wide and a short PR interval is present, the block is probably type II.

Keep in mind that type II block is more likely to impair cardiac output, lead to symptoms such as syncope, and progress to a more severe form of block. Be sure to monitor the patient carefully.

Cheat sheet

Signs of type II second-degree AV block

- *Atrial rhythm* — regular
- *Ventricular rhythm* — irregular if block is intermittent; regular if block is constant (such as 2:1 or 3:1)
- *PR interval* — constant for all conducted beats, prolonged in some cases
- *QRS complex* — usually wide

amination, you may note hypotension, and the pulse may be slow and regular or irregular.

How you intervene

If the dropped beats are infrequent and the patient shows no symptoms of decreased cardiac output, the doctor may choose only to observe the rhythm, particularly if the cause is thought to be reversible. If the patient is hypotensive, treatment aims to improve cardiac output by increasing the heart rate.

Because the conduction block occurs in the His-Purkinje system, transcutaneous pacing should be initiated quickly.

Pacemaker place

Type II second-degree AV block commonly requires placement of a pacemaker. A temporary pacemaker may be used until a permanent pacemaker can be placed.

When caring for a patient with type II second-degree block, assess his tolerance for the rhythm and the need for treatment to improve cardiac output. Evaluate for possible correctable causes such as ischemia.

Keep the patient on bed rest, if indicated, to reduce myocardial oxygen demands. Administer oxygen therapy as ordered. Observe the patient for progression to a more severe form of AV block. If the patient receives a pacemaker, teach him and his family about its use.

Bed rest may be necessary to reduce myocardial oxygen demands.

Third-degree AV block

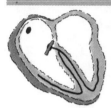

Also called complete heart block, third-degree AV block occurs when impulses from the atria are completely blocked at the AV node and can't be conducted to the ventricles. Maintaining our doorway analogy, this form of block is like a line of people waiting to go through a doorway, but no one can go through.

Beats of different drummers

Acting independently, the atria, generally under the control of the SA node, tend to maintain a regular rate of 60 to 100 beats/minute. The ventricular rhythm can originate from the AV node and maintain a rate of 40 to 60 beats/minute or from the Purkinje system in the ventricles and maintain a rate of 20 to 40 beats/minute.

The rhythm strip will look like a strip of P waves laid independently over a strip of QRS complexes. Note that the P wave doesn't conduct the QRS complex that follows it.

How it happens

Third-degree AV block that originates at the level of the AV node is most commonly a congenital condition. This block may also be caused by coronary artery disease, an anterior- or inferior-wall MI, degenerative changes in the heart, digoxin toxicity, calcium channel blockers, beta-adrenergic blockers, or surgical injury. It may be temporary or permanent.

Because the ventricular rate is so slow, third-degree AV block presents a potentially life-threatening situation because cardiac output can drop dramatically. In addition, the patient loses his atrial kick — that extra 30% of blood flow pushed into the ventricles by atrial contraction. That happens as a result of the loss of synchrony between the atrial and ventricular contractions. The loss of atrial kick further decreases cardiac output. Any exertion on the part of the patient can worsen symptoms.

What to look for

When analyzing an ECG for this rhythm, you'll note that the atrial and ventricular rhythms are regular. The P and R waves can be walked out across the strip, meaning that they appear to march across the strip in rhythm. (See *Identifying third-degree AV block,* page 160.)

Don't skip this strip

Identifying third-degree AV block

The following rhythm strip shows third-degree AV block. Look for these distinguishing characteristics.

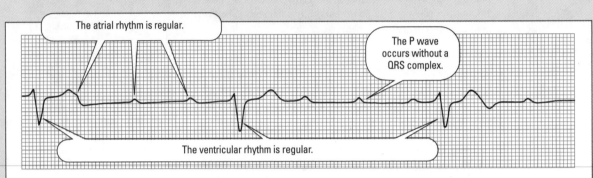

The atrial rhythm is regular.

The P wave occurs without a QRS complex.

The ventricular rhythm is regular.

- *Rhythm:* regular
- *Rate:* atrial 90 beats/minute; ventricular 30 beats/minute

- *P wave:* normal
- *PR interval:* varies
- *QRS complex:* 0.16 second

- *T wave:* normal
- *QT interval:* 0.56 second
- *Other:* none

Some P waves may be buried in QRS complexes or T waves. The PR interval will vary with no pattern or regularity. If the resulting rhythm, called the escape rhythm, originates in the AV node, the QRS complex will be normal and the ventricular rate will be 40 to 60 beats/minute. If the escape rhythm originates in the Purkinje system, the QRS complex will be wide, with a ventricular rate below 40 beats/minute.

Escape!

The PR interval varies because the atria and ventricles beat independently of each other. The QRS complex is determined by the site of the escape rhythm. Usually, the duration and configuration are normal; however, with an idioventricular escape rhythm (an escape rhythm originating in the ventricles), the duration is greater than 0.12 second and the complex is distorted.

While atrial and ventricular rates can vary with third-degree block, they're nearly the same with complete AV dissociation, a similar rhythm. (See *Complete AV dissociation,* page 162.)

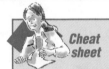

Cheat sheet

Signs of third-degree AV block

- *Atrial and ventricular rhythm*—regular
- *PR interval*—varies, with no regularity
- *P and R waves*—march across strip in rhythm; some P waves may be buried in QRS complexes or T waves

Serious signs and symptoms

Most patients with third-degree AV block experience significant symptoms, including severe fatigue, dyspnea, chest pain, light-headedness, changes in mental status, and loss of consciousness. You may note hypotension, pallor, diaphoresis, bradycardia, and a variation in the intensity of the pulse.

A few patients will be relatively free from symptoms, complaining only that they can't tolerate exercise and that they're often tired for no apparent reason. The severity of symptoms depends to a great extent on the resulting ventricular rate.

How you intervene

If cardiac output isn't adequate or the patient's condition seems to be deteriorating, therapy aims to improve the ventricular rate. Atropine may be given, or a temporary pacemaker may be used to restore adequate cardiac output.

Temporary pacing may be required until the cause of the block resolves or until a permanent pacemaker can be inserted. A permanent block requires placement of a permanent pacemaker. (See *Treating third-degree AV block.*)

Bundles of troubles

The patient with an anterior wall MI is more likely to have permanent third-degree AV block if the MI involved the bundle of His or the bundle branches than if it involved other areas of the myocardium. Those patients commonly require prompt placement of a permanent pacemaker.

An AV block in a patient with an inferior wall MI is more likely to be temporary, as a result of injury to the AV node. Placement of a permanent pacemaker is often delayed in such cases to evaluate recovery of the conduction system.

Check it out...

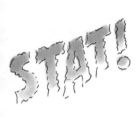

When caring for a patient with third-degree heart block, immediately assess the patient's tolerance of the rhythm and the need for treatment to support cardiac output and relieve symptoms. Make sure the patient has a patent I.V. line. Administer oxygen therapy as ordered. Evaluate for possible correctable causes of the arrhythmia, such as medications or ischemia. Minimize the patient's activity and maintain his bed rest.

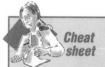

Cheat sheet

Escape rhythm

• *Originating in AV node* — normal QRS complex; ventricular rate of 40 to 60 beats/minute
• *Originating in Purkinje system* — wide QRS complex; ventricular rate below 40 beats/minute
• *PR interval* — unmeasurable
• *QRS complex* — usually normal; with idioventricular escape rhythm, duration greater than 0.12 second and distorted complex

I can't waste time

Treating third-degree AV block

• Atropine may be given.
• Temporary pacemaker may be used to restore cardiac output.
• Temporary pacing may be required until cause of block resolves or until permanent pacemaker can be inserted.

Don't skip this strip

Complete AV dissociation

With both third-degree atrioventricular (AV) block and complete AV dissociation, the atria and ventricles beat independently, each controlled by its own pacemaker. However, here's the key difference: In third-degree AV block, the atrial rate is faster than the ventricular rate. With complete AV dissociation, the two rates are usually about the same, with the ventricular rate slightly faster.

Rhythm disturbances

Never the primary problem, complete AV dissociation results from one of three underlying rhythm disturbances:

- slowed or impaired sinus impulse formation or SA conduction, as in sinus bradycardia or sinus arrest
- accelerated impulse formation in the AV junction or the ventricular pacemaker, as in junctional or ventricular tachycardia
- AV conduction disturbance, as in complete AV block.

When to treat

The clinical significance of complete AV dissociation—as well as treatment for the arrhythmia—depends on the underlying cause and its effects on the patient. If the underlying rhythm decreases cardiac output, the patient will need treatment to correct the arrhythmia.

Depending on the underlying cause, the patient may be treated with an antiarrhythmic, such as atropine or isoproterenol, to restore synchrony. Or the patient may be given a pacemaker to support a slow ventricular rate. If drug toxicity caused the original disturbance, the drug should be discontinued.

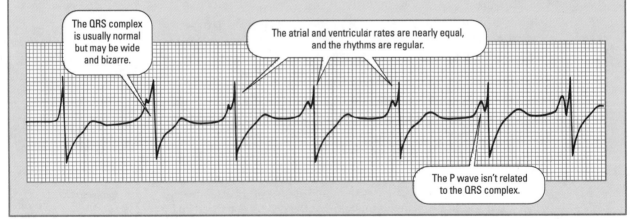

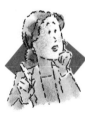

Quick quiz

1. No treatment is necessary if the patient has the form of AV block known as:
- A. first-degree AV block.
- B. type II second-degree AV block.
- C. third-degree AV block.

Answer: A. A patient with first-degree AV block rarely experiences symptoms and usually requires only monitoring for progression of the block.

2. In type I second-degree AV block, the PR interval:
- A. varies according to the ventricular response rate.
- B. progressively lengthens until a QRS complex is dropped.
- C. remains constant despite an irregular ventricular rhythm.

Answer: B. Progressive lengthening of the PR interval creates an irregular ventricular rhythm with a repeating pattern of groups of QRS complexes. Those groups are followed by a dropped beat in which the P wave isn't followed by a QRS complex.

3. Myocardial ischemia may cause cells in the AV node to repolarize:
- A. normally.
- B. faster than normal.
- C. more slowly than normal.

Answer: C. Injured cells conduct impulses slowly or inconsistently. Relief of the ischemia can restore normal function to the AV node.

4. Type II second-degree block is generally considered more serious than type I because in most cases of type II the:
- A. cardiac output is diminished.
- B. ventricular rate rises above 100 beats/minute.
- C. peripheral vascular system shuts down almost as soon as the arrhythmia begins.

Answer: A. This form of AV block causes a decrease in cardiac output, particularly if the sinus rhythm is slow and the ratio of conducted beats to dropped beats is low such as 2:1.

5. AV block can be caused by inadvertent damage to the heart's conduction system during cardiac surgery. Damage is most likely to occur in surgery involving which area of the heart?

    A.   Pulmonic valve

    B.   Mitral valve

    C.   Aortic valve

Answer: B. AV block can be caused by surgery involving the mitral or tricuspid valve or in the closure of a ventricular septal defect.

6. A main component of the treatment for third-degree AV block is:

    A.   use of a pacemaker.

    B.   administration of calcium channel blockers.

    C.   administration of oxygen and antiarrhythmics.

Answer: B. Temporary pacing may be required for this rhythm disturbance until the cause of the block resolves or until a permanent pacemaker can be implanted. Permanent third-degree AV block requires placement of a permanent pacemaker.

7. Treatment of first-degree AV block is aimed at correcting the underlying cause. Which of the following may cause first-degree AV block?

    A.   Stress

    B.   Digoxin

    C.   Angiotensin-converting enzyme inhibitors

Answer: B. First-degree AV block may be caused by myocardial infarction or ischemia, myocarditis, degenerative changes in the heart, and such medications as digoxin, calcium channel blockers, and beta-adrenergic blockers.

Way to go! Now try the test strips on the next page.

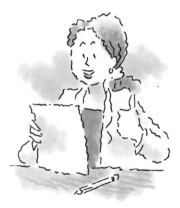

Test strips

OK, try a few test strips. Answer the question accompanying each strip; then check your answers with ours.

8. In the rhythm strip that follows, the atrial and ventricular rhythms are regular; both rates are 75 beats/minute; the P wave is of normal size and configuration; the PR interval is 0.34 second; the QRS complex is 0.08 second; the T wave is of normal configuration; and the QT interval is 0.42 second. You would identify the rhythm as:

    A.   type II second-degree AV block.
    B.   third-degree AV block.
    C.   first-degree AV block.

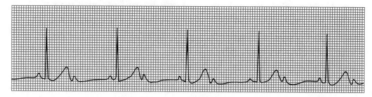

Answer: C. This strip shows sinus rhythm with first-degree AV block.

9. In the following ECG strip, the atrial and ventricular rhythms are regular; the atrial rate is 100 beats/minute; the ventricular rate is 50 beats/minute; the P wave is of normal size and configuration; the PR interval is 0.14 second; the QRS complex is 0.06 second; the T wave is of normal configuration; and the QT interval is 0.44 second. You would identify the rhythm as:

    A.   type I second-degree AV block.
    B.   type II second-degree AV block.
    C.   third-degree AV block.

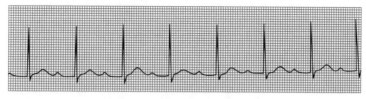

Answer: B. This strip shows type II second-degree AV block.

10. You would identify the rhythm in this strip as:
A.   first-degree AV block.
B.   type I second-degree AV block.
C.   third-degree AV block.

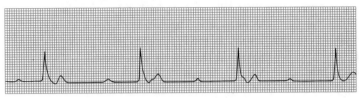

Answer: C. The atrial and ventricular rhythms are regular; the atrial rate is 75 beats/minute; the ventricular rate is 36 beats/minute; the P wave is of normal size and configuration, with no relation to the QRS complex; the QRS complex is 0.16 second, wide, and bizarre; the T wave is of normal configuration, except for the second beat, which is distorted by a P wave; and the QT interval is 0.42 second. These observations indicate third-degree AV block.

Scoring

☆☆☆   If you answered all ten questions correctly, way to go! You're clearly Ruler of Noble Node!

☆☆   If you answered seven to nine questions correctly, excellent! You're a Royal Knight of Noble Node!

☆   If you answered fewer than seven questions correctly, that's OK. You're Most High Sheriff of Noble Node!

Part III

Treating arrhythmias

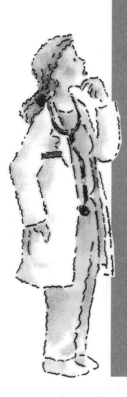

9

Pacemakers

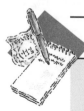

Just the facts

This chapter provides an overview of pacemakers and will help you recognize malfunctions and respond to them quickly. In this chapter, you'll learn:

♦ what a pacemaker is, what its components are, and how it works

♦ what kinds of pacemakers are available, how they're classified, and how they affect ECG tracings

♦ how to detect, identify, and correct pacemaker malfunctions

♦ how to care for a patient with a pacemaker

♦ what to teach patients about pacemakers.

A look at pacemakers

A pacemaker is an artificial device that electrically stimulates the myocardium to depolarize, which begins a contraction.

Pacemakers may be used when a patient has an arrhythmia, such as certain bradyarrhythmias and tachyarrhythmias, sick sinus syndrome, or atrioventricular (AV) blocks. The device may be temporary or permanent, depending on the patient's condition. Frequently, pacemakers are necessary following myocardial infarction or cardiac surgery.

Keeping the beat going

Pacemakers work by generating an impulse from a power source and transmitting that impulse to the heart muscle. The impulse flows throughout the heart and causes the heart muscle to depolarize. Pacemakers consist of three components: the pulse generator, the pacing leads, and the electrode tip.

Making the pacer work

The pulse generator contains the pacemaker's power source and circuitry. The lithium batteries in a permanent or implanted pacemaker are its power source and last about 10 years. The circuitry of the pacemaker is a microchip that guides heart pacing.

A temporary pacemaker, which isn't implanted, is about the size of a small radio or a telemetry box and is powered by alkaline batteries. These units also contain a microchip and are programmed by a touch pad or dials.

A look at pacing leads

Pacing leads have either one electrode (unipolar) or two (bipolar). These illustrations show the difference between the two leads.

Unipolar lead
In a unipolar system, electrical current moves from the pulse generator through the leadwire to the negative pole. From there, it stimulates the heart and returns to the pulse generator's metal surface (the positive pole) to complete the circuit.

Bipolar lead
In a bipolar system, current flows from the pulse generator through the leadwire to the negative pole at the tip. At that point, it stimulates the heart and then flows back to the positive pole to complete the circuit.

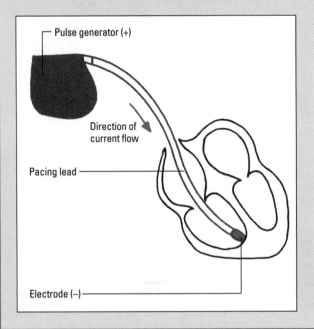

Pulse generator (+)

Direction of current flow

Pacing lead

Electrode (–)

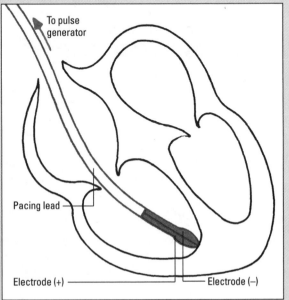

To pulse generator

Pacing lead

Electrode (+)

Electrode (–)

A stimulus on the move

An electrical stimulus from the pulse generator moves through wires or pacing leads to the electrode tips. The leads for a pacemaker designed to stimulate a single heart chamber are placed in either the atrium or the ventricle. For dual-chamber, or AV, pacing, the leads are placed in both chambers, usually on the right side of the heart.

Generating the impulse

The electrodes—one on a unipolar lead or two on a bipolar lead—send information about electrical impulses in the myocardium back to the pulse generator. The pulse generator senses the heart's electrical activity and responds according to how it's been programmed.

A unipolar lead system is more sensitive to the heart's intrinsic electrical activity than is a bipolar system. A bipolar system isn't as easily affected by electrical activity outside the heart and the generator (for example, from skeletal muscle contraction or magnetic fields). A bipolar system is more difficult to implant, however. (See *A look at pacing leads.*)

Working with pacemakers

On an ECG, you'll notice a pacemaker spike right away. (See *Pacemaker spikes.*) It occurs when the pacemaker sends an electrical impulse to the heart muscle. That impulse appears as a vertical line or spike.

Depending on the position of the electrode, the spike appears in different locations on the waveform.

• When the atria are stimulated by the pacemaker, the spike is followed by a P wave and the patient's baseline QRS complex and T wave. This series of waveforms represents successful pacing, or capture, of the myocardium. The P wave may look different from the patient's normal P wave.

• When the ventricles are stimulated by a pacemaker, the spike is followed by a QRS complex and a T wave. The QRS complex appears wider than the patient's own QRS complex because of the way the ventricles are depolarized.

• When the pacemaker stimulates both the atria and the ventricles, the spike is followed by a P wave, then a spike, and then a QRS complex. Be aware that the type of pacemaker used and the patient's condition may affect whether every beat is paced.

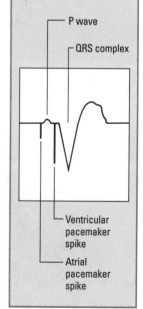

Pacemaker spikes

Pacemaker impulses—the stimuli that travel from the pacemaker to the heart—are visible on the patient's ECG tracing as spikes. Large or small, pacemaker spikes appear above or below the isoelectric line. This example shows an atrial and a ventricular pacemaker spike.

P wave

QRS complex

Ventricular pacemaker spike

Atrial pacemaker spike

Permanent and temporary pacemakers

Depending on the patient's signs and symptoms, a permanent or a temporary pacemaker can be used to maintain heart rhythm. Lead placement varies according to the patient's specific needs.

Permanent pacemakers

A permanent pacemaker is used to treat chronic heart conditions such as AV block. It's surgically implanted, usually under local anesthesia. The leads are placed transvenously, positioned in the appropriate chambers, and then anchored to the endocardium. (See *Placing a permanent pacemaker.*)

Pocket generator

The generator is then implanted in a pocket made from subcutaneous tissue. The pocket is usually constructed under the clavicle. Most permanent pacemakers are programmed before implantation. The programming sets the conditions under which the pacemaker functions and can be adjusted externally if necessary.

Temporary pacemakers

A temporary pacemaker is often inserted in an emergency. The patient may show signs of decreased cardiac output, such as hypotension or syncope. The temporary pacemaker supports the patient until the condition resolves.

A temporary pacemaker can also serve as a bridge until a permanent pacemaker is inserted. Temporary pacemakers are used for patients with low-grade heart block, bradycardia, or low cardiac output. Several types of temporary pacemakers are available, including transvenous, epicardial, and transcutaneous.

Going the transvenous way

Doctors may use the transvenous approach — inserting the pacemaker through a vein, such as the subclavian or internal jugular vein — when inserting a temporary pacemaker at the bedside or in other nonsurgical environments. The transvenous pacemaker is probably the most common and reliable type of temporary pacemaker. It's usually inserted at the bedside or in a fluoroscopy suite. The leadwires are advanced through a catheter into the right ventricle or atrium and then connected to the pulse generator.

Taking the epicardial route

Epicardial pacemakers are commonly used for patients undergoing cardiac surgery. The doctor attaches the tips of the leadwires to the surface of the heart and then brings the wires through the

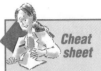
Cheat sheet

Atrial and ventricular stimulation

• *Atria:* spike followed by a P wave and the patient's baseline QRS complex and T wave
• *Ventricles:* spike followed by a QRS complex and T wave
• *Atria and ventricles:* spike followed by a P wave, then a spike, and then a QRS complex

Placing a permanent pacemaker

The surgeon who implants the endocardial pacemaker usually selects a transvenous route and begins lead placement by inserting a catheter percutaneously or by venous cutdown. Then, with a stylet and fluoroscopic guidance, the surgeon threads the catheter through the vein until the tip reaches the endocardium.

Atrial lead

For lead placement in the atrium, the tip must lodge in the right atrium or coronary sinus, as shown here. For placement in the ventricle, it must lodge within the right ventricular apex in one of the interior muscular ridges, or trabeculae.

Implanting the generator

When the lead is in the proper position, the surgeon secures the pulse generator in a subcutaneous pocket of tissue just below the clavicle. Changing the generator's battery or microchip circuitry requires only a shallow incision over the site and a quick component exchange.

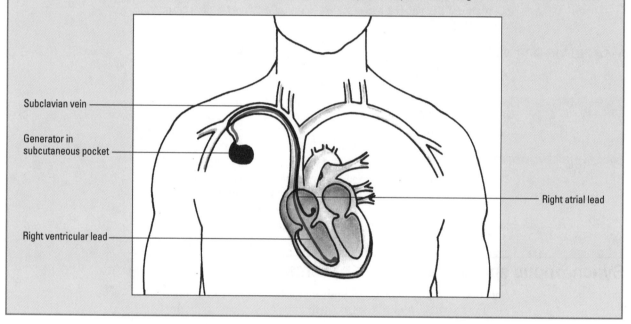

chest wall, below the incision. They're then attached to the pulse generator. The leadwires are usually removed several days after surgery or when the patient no longer requires them.

Following the transcutaneous path

Use of an external or transcutaneous pacemaker has become commonplace in the past several years. In this noninvasive method, one electrode is placed on the patient's anterior chest wall, and a second is applied to his back. An external pulse generator then emits pacing impulses that travel through the skin to the heart muscle.

Transcutaneous pacing is a quick and effective method of pacing the heart rhythm and is often used in emergencies until a transvenous pacemaker can be inserted. However, some alert patients can't tolerate the irritating sensations produced from prolonged pacing at the levels needed to pace the heart externally.

Setting the controls

When your patient has a temporary pacemaker, you'll notice several types of settings on the pulse generator. The rate control regulates how many impulses are generated in 1 minute and is measured in pulses per minute (ppm). The rate is usually set at 60 to 80 ppm. (See *A look at a pulse generator.*) The pacemaker fires if the patient's heart rate falls below the preset rate. The rate may be set higher if the patient has a tachyarrhythmia that's being treated with overdrive pacing.

Measuring the output

The electrical output of a pacemaker is measured in milliamperes. This measurement represents the stimulation threshold, or how much energy is required to stimulate the cardiac muscle to depolarize. The stimulation threshold is sometimes referred to as the energy required for capture.

Sensing the norm

You can also program the pacemaker's sensing threshold, measured in millivolts. Most pacemakers let the heart function naturally and assist only when necessary. The sensing threshold allows the pacemaker to do this by sensing the heart's normal activity.

Synchronous and asynchronous pacemakers

Pacemakers can also be classified according to how they stimulate the heart. A synchronous, or demand, pacemaker responds to the heart's activity by monitoring the intrinsic rhythm and pacing only when the heart can't do so itself. An asynchronous, or fixed rate, pacemaker fires at a preset heart rate regardless of the heart's intrinsic cycle. This type of pacemaker is rarely used.

Pacemaker codes

The capabilities of pacemakers may be described by a five-letter coding system, although three letters more commonly are used. (See *Pacemaker coding system,* page 176.)

A look at a pulse generator

Below is an illustration of a single-chamber temporary pulse generator with brief descriptions of its various parts.

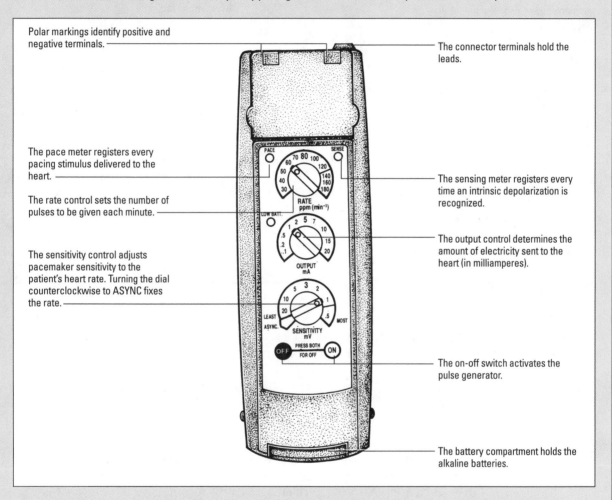

Polar markings identify positive and negative terminals.

The pace meter registers every pacing stimulus delivered to the heart.

The rate control sets the number of pulses to be given each minute.

The sensitivity control adjusts pacemaker sensitivity to the patient's heart rate. Turning the dial counterclockwise to ASYNC fixes the rate.

The connector terminals hold the leads.

The sensing meter registers every time an intrinsic depolarization is recognized.

The output control determines the amount of electricity sent to the heart (in milliamperes).

The on-off switch activates the pulse generator.

The battery compartment holds the alkaline batteries.

Introducing letter 1

The first letter of the code identifies the heart chambers being paced. These are the options and the letters used to signify those options:
- V = Ventricle
- A = Atrium
- D = Dual (ventricle and atrium)
- O = None.

Pacemaker coding system

A coding system for pacemaker functions can provide a simple description of pacemaker capabilities. One commonly used coding system employs three letters to describe functions.

The first letter refers to the chamber paced by the pacemaker. The second refers to the chamber sensed by the pacemaker. The third refers to the pacemaker's response to the sensed event.

In the example shown here, both chambers (represented in the code by *D,* for dual) are paced and sensed, and the pacemaker responds by firing impulses to both chambers.

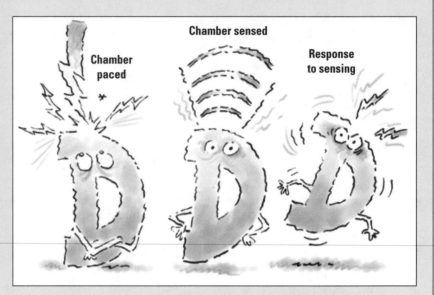

Chamber paced   **Chamber sensed**   **Response to sensing**

Learning about letter 2

The second letter of the code signifies the heart chamber in which the pacemaker senses the intrinsic activity:
- V = Ventricle
- A = Atrium
- D = Dual (ventricle and atrium)
- O = None.

Looking at letter 3

The third letter shows the pacemaker's response to the intrinsic electrical activity it senses in the atrium or ventricle:
- T = Triggers pacing (For instance, if atrial activity is sensed, ventricular pacing may be triggered.)
- I = Inhibits pacing (If the pacemaker senses intrinsic activity, it won't fire.)
- D = Dual (The pacemaker can be triggered or inhibited depending on the mode and where intrinsic activity occurs.)
- O = None. (The pacemaker doesn't change its mode in response to sensed activity.)

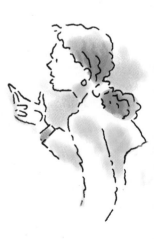

Figuring out letter 4

The fourth letter of the code describes the pacemaker's programmability; the letter tells whether an external programming device can modify the pacemaker:
- P = Programmable basic functions
- M = Multiprogrammable parameters
- C = Communicating functions (such as telemetry)
- R = Rate responsiveness (The rate adjusts to fit the patient's metabolic needs and achieve normal hemodynamic status.)
- O = None.

Last but not least, letter 5

The final letter of the code refers to the pacemaker's response to a tachyarrhythmia:
- P = Pacing ability (The pacemaker's rapid bursts pace the heart at a rate above its intrinsic rate to override the source of tachycardia. When the stimulation ceases, the tachyarrhythmia breaks. Increased arrhythmia may result.)
- S = Shock (An implantable cardioverter-defibrillator identifies ventricular tachycardia and delivers a shock to stop the arrhythmia.)
- D = Dual ability to shock and pace
- O = None.

Pacemaker modes

The mode of a pacemaker indicates its functions. Several different modes may be used during pacing, and they may or may not mimic the normal cardiac cycle. Here are four of the more commonly used modes and their three-letter abbreviations. (A three-letter code, rather than a five-letter code, is typically used to describe pacemaker function.)

AAI mode

The AAI, or atrial demand, pacemaker is a single-chambered pacemaker that paces and senses the atria. When the pacemaker senses intrinsic atrial activity, it inhibits pacing and resets itself. Only the atria are paced.

Not in block or brady

Because AAI pacemakers require a functioning AV node and ventricular conduction, they aren't used in AV block or ventricular bradycardia. An AAI pacemaker may be used in patients with sinus bradycardia, which may occur after cardiac surgery, or with

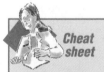

Cheat sheet

Pacemaker modes

- *AAI:* single-chambered pacemaker; paces and senses the atria
- *VVI:* paces and senses the ventricles
- *DVI:* paces both the atria and ventricles
- *DDD:* fires when ventricle doesn't respond on its own; paces the atria when atrial rate falls below the lower set rate

sick sinus syndrome as long as the His-Purkinje system isn't diseased.

VVI mode

The VVI, or ventricular demand, pacemaker paces and senses the ventricles. (See *AAI and VVI pacemakers.*) When it senses intrinsic ventricular activity, it inhibits pacing. This single-chambered

---

AAI and VVI pacemakers

Both an AAI and a VVI pacemaker are single-chamber pacemakers. The electrode for an AAI is placed in the atrium; the electrode for a VVI is placed in the ventricle. These rhythm strips show how each pacemaker works.

AAI pacemaker
Note how the AAI pacemaker senses and paces the atria only. The QRS complex that follows occurs as a result of the heart's own conduction.

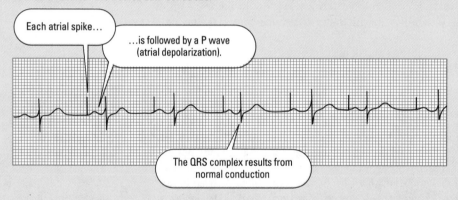

Each atrial spike...

...is followed by a P wave (atrial depolarization).

The QRS complex results from normal conduction

VVI pacemaker
The VVI pacemaker senses and paces the ventricles. When each spike is followed by a depolarization, as shown here, the rhythm is said to reflect 100% capture.

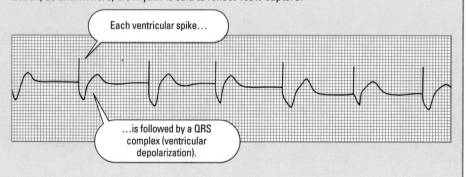

Each ventricular spike...

...is followed by a QRS complex (ventricular depolarization).

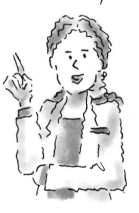

These rhythm strips show how AAI and VVI pacemakers work.

pacemaker benefits patients with complete heart block and those needing intermittent pacing. Because it doesn't affect atrial activity, it's used for patients who don't need an atrial kick — the extra 15% to 30% of cardiac output that comes from atrial contraction.

Unsynchronized activity

If the patient has spontaneous atrial activity, the VVI pacemaker won't synchronize the ventricular activity with it, so tricuspid and mitral regurgitation may develop. Sedentary patients may receive this pacemaker, but it won't adjust its rate for more active patients.

DVI mode

The DVI, or AV sequential, pacemaker paces both the atria and ventricles. (See *DVI pacemaker rhythm strip*.) However, this dual-chambered pacemaker senses only the ventricles' intrinsic activity, inhibiting its pacing there.

Two types of DVI pacemakers are used:
• The committed DVI pacemaker doesn't sense intrinsic activity during the AV interval — the time between an atrial and ventricular spike. It generates an impulse even with spontaneous ventricular depolarization.

DVI pacemaker rhythm strip

Here's an ECG tracing from a committed DVI pacemaker, which paces both the atria and the ventricles. The pacemaker senses ventricular activity only. In two of the complexes, the pacemaker didn't sense the intrinsic QRS complex because the complex occurred during the AV interval, when the pacemaker was already committed to fire.

With a noncommitted DVI pacemaker, spikes after the QRS complex wouldn't appear because the stimulus to pace the ventricles would be inhibited.

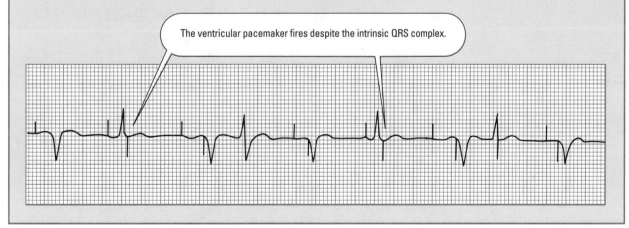

The ventricular pacemaker fires despite the intrinsic QRS complex.

• The noncommitted DVI pacemaker is inhibited if a spontaneous depolarization occurs within the AV interval.

Who is helped

The DVI pacemaker helps patients with AV block or sick sinus syndrome who have a diseased His-Purkinje conduction system. It provides the benefits of AV synchrony and atrial kick, thus improving cardiac output. However, it can't vary the atrial rate and isn't helpful in atrial fibrillation because it can't capture the atria. In addition, it may needlessly fire or inhibit its own pacing.

DDD mode

A DDD or universal pacemaker is used with severe AV block. (See *DDD pacemaker rhythm strip.*) However, because the pacemaker possesses so many capabilities, it may be hard to troubleshoot problems. Its advantages include its:
• versatility
• programmability
• ability to change modes automatically

DDD pacemaker rhythm strip

On this DDD pacemaker rhythm strip, complexes 1, 2, 4, and 7 reveal the atrial-synchronous mode, set at a rate of 70. The patient has an intrinsic P wave; the pacemaker serves only to make sure the ventricles respond.

Complexes 3, 5, 8, 10, and 12 are intrinsic ventricular depolarizations. The pacemaker senses these depolarizations and inhibits firing. In complexes 6, 9, and 11, the pacemaker is pacing both the atria and the ventricles in sequence. In complex 13, only the atria are paced; the ventricles respond on their own.

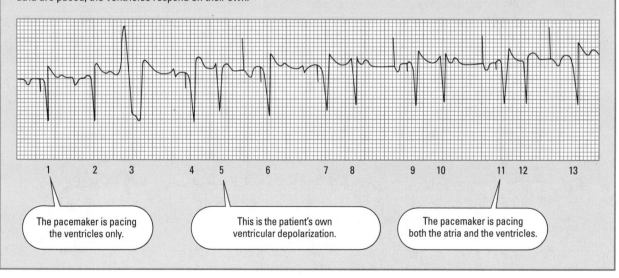

The pacemaker is pacing the ventricles only.

This is the patient's own ventricular depolarization.

The pacemaker is pacing both the atria and the ventricles.

• ability to mimic the normal physiologic cardiac cycle, maintaining AV synchrony
• ability to sense and pace the atria and ventricles at the same time according to the intrinsic atrial rate and the maximal rate limit.

Home, home on the rate range

Unlike other pacemakers, the DDD pacemaker is set with a rate range, rather than a single critical rate. It senses atrial activity and ensures that the ventricles respond to each atrial stimulation, thereby maintaining normal AV synchrony.

Firing and pacing

The DDD pacemaker fires when the ventricle doesn't respond on its own, and it paces the atria when the atrial rate falls below the lower set rate. (See *Evaluating a DDD pacemaker rhythm strip.*) In a patient with a high atrial rate, a safety mechanism allows the pacemaker to follow the intrinsic atrial rate only as far as a preset upper limit. That limit is usually set at about 130 beats/minute and helps to prevent the ventricles from following atrial tachycardia or atrial flutter.

Evaluating pacemakers

Now you're ready to find out if your patient's pacemaker is working correctly. To do this, follow the procedure described below.

1. Read the records

First, determine the pacemaker's mode and settings. If your patient had a permanent pacemaker implanted before admission, ask him if he has a wallet card from the manufacturer that notes the mode and settings.

If the pacemaker was recently implanted, check the patient's records for information. Don't check only the ECG tracing — you might misinterpret it if you don't know the pacemaker type. For instance, if the tracing has ventricular spikes but no atrial spikes, you might guess that it's a VVI pacemaker when it's actually a DVI pacemaker that has lost its atrial output.

2. Look at the leads

Next, review the patient's 12-lead ECG. If it isn't available, examine lead V_1 or MCL_1 instead. Invert the QRS complex here, just as with a left bundle-branch block. An upright QRS complex may mean that the leadwire is out of position, perhaps even perforating the septum and lodging in the left ventricle.

Evaluating a DDD pacemaker rhythm strip

Look for these possible events when examining a rhythm strip showing the activities of a DDD pacemaker.
• Intrinsic rhythm: No pacemaker activity occurs because none is needed.
• Intrinsic P wave followed by a ventricular pacemaker spike: The pacemaker is tracking the atrial rate and assuring a ventricular response.
• Pacemaker spike before a P wave, then an intrinsic ventricular QRS complex: The atrial rate is falling below the lower rate limit, causing the atrial channel to fire. Normal conduction to the ventricles then ensues.
• Pacemaker spike before a P wave and a pacemaker spike before the QRS complex: No intrinsic activity occurs in either the atria or the ventricles.

3. Scrutinize the spikes

Then select a monitoring lead that clearly shows the pacemaker spikes. Make sure the lead you select doesn't cause the cardiac monitor to mistake a spike for a QRS complex, and then double-count the heart rate monitor. This may cause the alarm to go off, falsely signaling a high heart rate.

4. Mull over the mode

When looking at the ECG tracing of a patient with a pacemaker, consider the pacemaker mode. Then interpret the paced rhythm. Does it match what you know about the pacemaker?

5. Unravel the rhythm

Look for information that tells you which chamber is paced. Is there capture? Is there a P wave or QRS complex after each atrial or ventricular spike? Or do the P waves and QRS complexes stem from intrinsic activity?

Look for information about the pacemaker's sensing ability. If intrinsic atrial or ventricular activity is present, what is the pacemaker's response? Look at the rate. What is the pacing rate per minute? Is it appropriate given the pacemaker settings? Although you can determine the rate quickly by counting the number of complexes in a 6-second ECG strip, a more accurate method is to count the number of small boxes between complexes and divide this into 1,500.

Troubleshooting problems

Malfunction of a pacemaker can lead to arrhythmias, hypotension, and syncope. (See *When a pacemaker malfunctions.*) Common problems with pacemakers that can lead to low cardiac output and loss of AV synchrony include:
• failure to capture
• failure to pace
• undersensing
• oversensing.

Failure to capture

Failure to capture is indicated on an ECG by a pacemaker spike without the appropriate atrial or ventricular response — a spike without a complex. Think of failure to capture as the pacemaker's inability to stimulate the chamber.

Causes include acidosis, an electrolyte imbalance, fibrosis, an incorrect lead position, a low milliampere setting, depletion of the

Cheat sheet

Assessing pacemaker function

• First, determine pacemaker mode and settings.
• Next, review the patient's 12-lead ECG.
• Then select the monitoring lead that clearly shows pacemaker spikes.
• Then interpret paced rhythm.
• Look for information that tells which chamber is paced and for information about the pacemaker's sensing ability.

Mixed signals

When a pacemaker malfunctions

Occasionally, pacemakers fail to function properly. When that happens, you'll need to take immediate action to correct the problem. The strips shown below are examples of problems that can occur with a temporary pacemaker.

Failure to capture

• If the patient's condition has changed, notify the doctor and ask for new settings.

• If pacemaker settings have been altered by the patient or someone else, return them to their correct positions. Make sure the face of the pacemaker is covered with its plastic shield. Remind the patient not to touch the dials.

• If the heart still doesn't respond, carefully check all connections. You can also increase the milliampere setting slowly (according to your facility's policy or the doctor's orders), turn the patient from side to side, change the battery, or reverse the cables in the pulse generator so the positive wire is in the negative terminal and vice versa. Keep in mind that the doctor may order a chest X-ray to determine the position of the electrode.

Failure to pace

• If the pacing or indicator light flashes, check the connections to the cable and the position of the pacing electrode in the patient (done by X-ray).

• If the pulse generator is turned on but the indicators aren't flashing, change the battery. If that doesn't help, use a different pulse generator.

Failure to sense intrinsic beats

• If the pacemaker is undersensing (it fires but at the wrong times or for the wrong reasons), turn the sensitivity control completely to the right. If the pacemaker is oversensing (it incorrectly senses depolarization and refuses to fire when it should), turn the sensitivity control slightly to the left.

• Change the battery or pulse generator.

• Remove items in the room that might be causing electromechanical interference. Check that the bed is grounded. Unplug each piece of equipment, and then check to see if the interference stops.

• If the pacemaker is still firing on the T wave and all corrective actions have failed, turn off the pacemaker. Be sure atropine is available in case the patient's heart rate drops, and be prepared to initiate cardiopulmonary resuscitation if necessary.

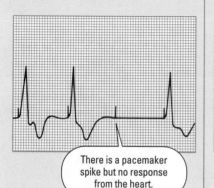

There is a pacemaker spike but no response from the heart.

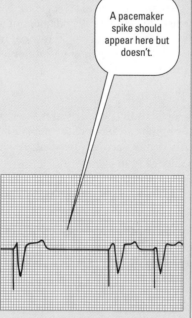

A pacemaker spike should appear here but doesn't.

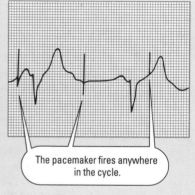

The pacemaker fires anywhere in the cycle.

battery, a broken or cracked leadwire, or perforation of the lead-wire through the myocardium.

Failure to pace

Failure to pace is indicated by no pacemaker activity on an ECG. The problem is caused by battery or circuit failure, cracked or broken leads, or interference between atrial and ventricular sensing in a dual-chambered pacemaker. It can lead to asystole.

Failure to sense

Undersensing is indicated by a pacemaker spike when intrinsic cardiac activity is already present. Think of it as help being given when none is needed. In asynchronous pacemakers that have codes such as VOO or DOO, undersensing is a programming limitation.

Spikes out of place

When undersensing occurs in synchronous pacemakers, spikes occur on the ECG where they shouldn't. Although they may appear in any part of the cardiac cycle, the spikes are especially dangerous if they fall on the T wave, where they can cause ventricular tachycardia or fibrillation.

In synchronous pacemakers, the problem is caused by electrolyte imbalances, disconnection or dislodgment of a lead, improper lead placement, increased sensing threshold from edema or fibrosis at the electrode tip, drug interactions, or a depleted or dead pacemaker battery.

Oversensing

If the pacemaker is too sensitive, it can misinterpret muscle movement or other events in the cardiac cycle as depolarization. Then it won't pace when the patient actually needs it, and heart rate and AV synchrony won't be maintained.

How you intervene

Make sure you're familiar with different types of pacemakers and how they function. This will save you time and worry during an emergency. When caring for a patient with a pacemaker, follow these guidelines.

Checks and balances

- Assist with pacemaker insertion as appropriate.
- Regularly check the patient's pacemaker settings, connections, and functions.
- Monitor the patient to see how well he tolerates the pacemaker.

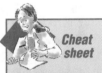

Cheat sheet

Trouble-shooting pacemakers

- *Failure to capture:* indicated by spike without a complex
- *Failure to pace:* no pacemaker activity on ECG
- *Undersensing:* help being given when none is needed
- *Oversensing:* won't pace when the patient actually needs it

• Reposition the patient with a temporary pacemaker carefully. Turning may dislodge the leadwire.
• Avoid potential microshocks to the patient by ensuring that electrical equipment is grounded properly, including the patient's bed.
• Remember that pacemaker spikes on the monitor don't mean your patient is stable. Be sure to check his vital signs and assess for signs and symptoms of decreased cardiac output, such as hypotension, chest pain, dyspnea, and syncope.

On the alert

• Be alert for signs of infection.
• Watch for subcutaneous air around the pacemaker insertion site. Subcutaneous tissue that contains air feels crunchy under your fingers.
• Look for pectoral muscle twitching or hiccups that occur in synchrony with the pacemaker. Both are signs of stimulation, which may be serious. Notify the doctor if you note any of those conditions.
• Watch for a perforated ventricle and cardiac tamponade. Signs and symptoms include persistent hiccups, distant heart sounds, pulsus paradoxus (a drop in the strength of a pulse during inspiration), hypotension with narrowed pulse pressure, cyanosis, distended neck veins, decreased urine output, restlessness, and complaints of fullness in the chest. Notify the doctor immediately if you note any of those signs and symptoms.

What to teach the patient

When a patient gets a pacemaker, be sure to cover these points:
• Explain to the patient and family why a pacemaker is needed, how it works, and what they can expect.
• Warn the patient with a temporary pacemaker not to get out of bed without assistance.
• Warn the patient with a transcutaneous pacemaker to expect twitching of the pectoral muscles. Reassure him that he'll receive medication if he can't tolerate the discomfort.
• Instruct the patient not to manipulate the pacemaker wires or pulse generator.
• Give the patient with a permanent pacemaker the manufacturer's identification card, and tell him to carry it at all times.
• Teach the patient and family how to care for the incision, how to take a pulse, and what to do if the pulse drops below the pacemaker rate.
• Advise the patient to avoid tight clothing or other direct pressure over the pulse generator, to avoid magnetic resonance imag-

> A patient who gets a pacemaker needs to be educated about its use.

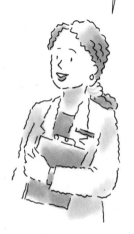

ing scans and certain other diagnostic studies, and to notify the doctor if he feels confused, light-headed, or short of breath. The patient should also notify the doctor if he has palpitations, hiccups, or a rapid or unusually slow heart rate.

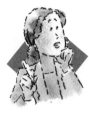

Quick quiz

1. When using an external temporary pacemaker, the energy level should be set at:
- A.   the highest milliampere setting the patient can tolerate.
- B.   the lowest milliampere setting that ensures capture of the myocardium.
- C.   a milliampere setting midway between the setting that causes capture of the myocardium and the setting at which symptoms first appear.

Answer: B. Select the lowest milliampere setting that causes capture of the myocardium. Higher energy levels will be too irritating for the patient.

2. When a VVI pacemaker senses intrinsic ventricular activity, it responds by:
- A.   inhibiting its pacing.
- B.   triggering its pacing.
- C.   doing nothing.

Answer: A. The third letter of the pacemaker code represents its response to ventricular activity. "I" stands for "inhibited."

3. Severe hiccups in a patient with a temporary transvenous pacemaker are probably due to:
- A.   movement of the pacemaker electrode.
- B.   the milliamperes being set too low.
- C.   tight clothing over the pulse generator.

Answer: A. Hiccups can be triggered by electrode movement, which can cause the pacemaker to stimulate the diaphragm. They can also result from the extracardiac stimulation caused by setting the milliamperes too high, not too low.

4. Failure to capture is represented on the ECG as:
- A.   no pacemaker activity.
- B.   spikes occurring where they shouldn't.
- C.   a spike without a complex.

Answer: C. A spike without a complex indicates the pacemaker's inability to capture or stimulate the chamber.

5. Decreased urine output and distant heart sounds in a patient with a recently implanted pacemaker indicate:
    A.   pacemaker failure.
    B.   cardiac tamponade.
    C.   myocardial infarction.

Answer: B. Decreased urine output and distant heart sounds indicate cardiac tamponade resulting from a perforated ventricle.

6. In a synchronous pacemaker, failure to sense is characterized on the ECG by:
    A.   lack of a pacemaker spike.
    B.   a pacemaker spike in the presence of intrinsic activity.
    C.   a pacemaker spike without evidence of cardiac stimulation.

Answer: B. Undersensing is indicated by a pacemaker spike when intrinsic cardiac activity is present.

Test strip

Time to try out a test strip. Ready? Go!

7. In the following ECG strip, the pacemaker is pacing and sensing the ventricles with 100% capture. The mode of response can't be evaluated because of lack of intrinsic activity. You would determine that the patient has a:
    A.   VVI pacemaker.
    B.   DVI pacemaker.
    C.   AAI pacemaker.

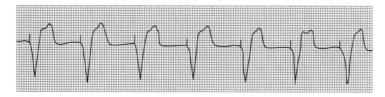

Answer: A. The patient has a VVI, or demand, pacemaker, which inhibits pacing when it senses ventricular activity.

8. The first letter in the five-letter coding system for pacemakers identifies the:
    A.   chamber in which the pacemaker senses intrinsic activity.
    B.   heart chamber being paced.
    C.   pacemaker's response to the intrinsic electrical activity.

Answer: B. The first letter identifies the heart chamber being paced, the second letter signifies the heart chamber that senses intrinsic activity, and the third letter shows the pacemaker's response to that activity.

Scoring

☆☆☆ If you answered all eight questions correctly, all right! You're the new leader of the Mighty Myocardial Power Sources!

☆☆ If you answered six or seven questions correctly, terrific! You're first runner-up for the Power Sources and destined to take the lead soon!

☆ If you answered fewer than six questions correctly, no sweat. You've been voted most likely to generate Power Source impulses!

Drugs that treat arrhythmias

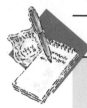

Just the facts

This chapter provides an overview of the antiarrhythmic drug classification system and specific drugs within each classification. In this chapter, you'll learn:

♦ how the antiarrhythmic classification system works

♦ what effects antiarrhythmics have on the cardiovascular and other body systems

♦ how to administer various antiarrhythmics and what their adverse effects are

♦ how to care for patients on antiarrhythmic drugs and what to teach them.

A look at antiarrhythmics

Almost half a million Americans die each year from cardiac arrhythmias; countless others suffer symptoms or lifestyle limitations. Along with other treatments, antiarrhythmic drugs can help alleviate symptoms and prolong life.

Antiarrhythmic drugs affect the movement of ions across the cell membrane and alter the electrophysiology of the cardiac cell. They're classified according to their effect on the cell's electrical activity (action potential) and their mechanism of action. (See *Antiarrhythmics and the action potential*, page 190.)

Drugs in the same class are similar in action and adverse effects. When you know where a particular drug fits in the classification system, you'll be better able to remember its actions and adverse effects.

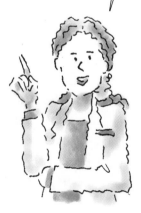

Antiarrhythmic drugs can help prolong life.

Antiarrhythmics and the action potential

Each class of antiarrhythmic drugs acts on a different phase of the action potential of the heart. Here's a rundown on the four classes of antiarrhythmics and how they affect action potential.

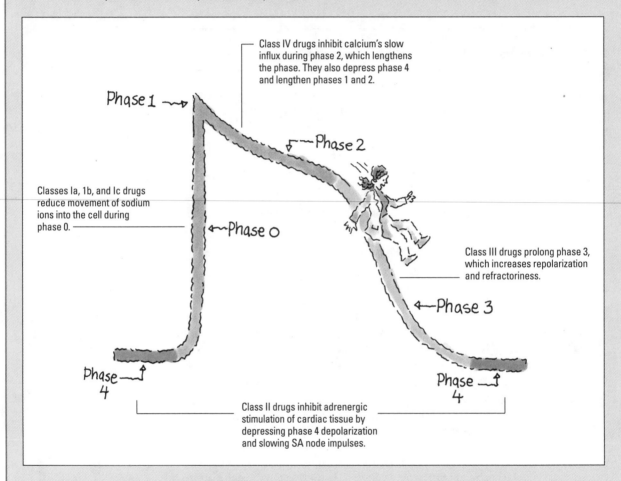

Class IV drugs inhibit calcium's slow influx during phase 2, which lengthens the phase. They also depress phase 4 and lengthen phases 1 and 2.

Phase 1

Phase 2

Classes Ia, 1b, and Ic drugs reduce movement of sodium ions into the cell during phase 0.

Phase 0

Class III drugs prolong phase 3, which increases repolarization and refractoriness.

Phase 3

Phase 4

Phase 4

Class II drugs inhibit adrenergic stimulation of cardiac tissue by depressing phase 4 depolarization and slowing SA node impulses.

Classifying antiarrhythmics

The classification system divides antiarrhythmic drugs into four major classes. Let's take a look at each one.

Class I blocks sodium

Class I drugs block the influx of sodium into the cell during phase 0 of the action potential. This minimizes the chance of sodium reaching its threshold potential and causing cells to depolarize.

Because phase 0 is also referred to as the sodium channel or fast channel, these drugs may also be called sodium channel blockers or fast channel blockers.

Antiarrhythmic drugs in this class are further categorized as:
• class Ia: reduce conductivity and prolong repolarization and the action potential
• class Ib: slow phase 0 depolarization, don't affect conductivity, and shorten phase 3 repolarization and the action potential
• class Ic: markedly slow phase 0 depolarization and reduce conduction, are used only for refractory arrhythmias, and are potentially proarrhythmic, meaning they can cause or worsen arrhythmias.

Class II blocks beta receptors

Class II drugs block sympathetic nervous system beta receptors and thereby decrease heart rate. Phase 4 depolarization is diminished depressing sinoatrial (SA) node automaticity and increasing atrial and atrioventricular (AV) nodal refractoriness, or resistance to stimulation.

Class III blocks potassium

Class III drugs are called potassium channel blockers because they block the movement of potassium during phase 3 of the action potential and prolong repolarization and the refractory period.

Class IV blocks calcium

Class IV drugs block the movement of calcium during phase 2 of the action potential. Because Phase 2 is also called the calcium channel or the slow channel, drugs that affect phase 2 are also known as calcium channel blockers or slow channel blockers. They prolong conductivity and increase the refractory period at the AV node.

Some drugs don't fit

Not all drugs fit neatly into those classifications. For example, sotalol possesses characteristics of both class II and class III drugs. Some drugs used to treat arrhythmias don't fit into the classification system at all. Those drugs include adenosine, digoxin, atropine, epinephrine, and magnesium. Despite these limitations, the classification system is helpful in understanding how antiarrhythmic drugs prevent and treat arrhythmias.

Drug distribution and clearance

Many patients receive antiarrhythmic drugs by I.V. bolus or infusion because they're more readily available that way than orally.

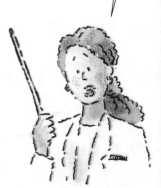

Some arrhythmias possess characteristics that don't fit into the classification system at all.

The cardiovascular system then distributes the drugs throughout the body, specifically to the site of action.

Most drugs are changed, or biotransformed, into active or inactive metabolites in the liver. The kidneys are the primary sites for the excretion of those metabolites. When administering these drugs, remember that patients with impaired heart, liver, or kidney function may suffer from inadequate drug effect or toxicity.

Antiarrhythmics by class

Broken down by classes, the following section describes commonly used antiarrhythmic drugs. It highlights their dosages, adverse effects, and recommendations for patient care.

Class Ia antiarrhythmics

Class Ia antiarrhythmic drugs are called sodium channel blockers. They include quinidine and procainamide. These drugs reduce the excitability of the cardiac cell, have an anticholinergic effect, and decrease cardiac contractility. Because the drugs prolong the QT

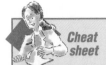

Cheat sheet

Class Ia antiarrhythmics

- Called sodium channel blockers
- Reduce excitability of cardiac cell
- Have anticholinergic effect
- Decrease cardiac contractility

Effects of class Ia antiarrhythmics

Class Ia antiarrhythmic drugs—including such drugs as quinidine and procainamide—affect the cardiac cycle in specific ways and lead to specific ECG changes, shown here. Class Ia antiarrhythmics:

- block sodium influx during phase 0, which depresses the rate of depolarization
- prolong repolarization and the duration of the action potential
- lengthen the refractory period
- decrease contractility.

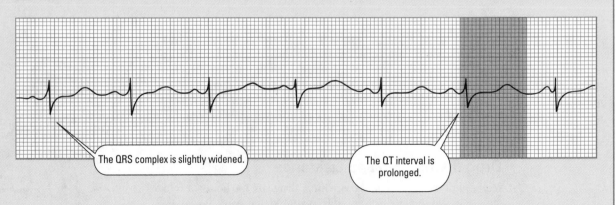

The QRS complex is slightly widened.

The QT interval is prolonged.

interval, the patient is prone to polymorphic ventricular tachycardia (VT). (See *Effects of class Ia antiarrhythmics.*)

Quinidine

Quinidine is used to treat patients with supraventricular and ventricular arrhythmias, such as atrial fibrillation or flutter, paroxysmal supraventricular tachycardia, and premature ventricular contractions (PVCs). The drug comes in several forms, including quinidine sulfate (Cin-Quin) and quinidine gluconate (Duraquin).

How to give it

Here's how to administer quinidine:
• To convert atrial flutter or fibrillation: 200 mg of quinidine sulfate orally every 2 to 3 hours for five to eight doses, with subsequent daily increases until sinus rhythm is restored or toxic effects develop.
• Initial dosage for paroxysmal supraventricular tachycardia: 400 to 600 mg of quinidine gluconate orally every 2 to 3 hours until sinus rhythm is restored or toxic effects develop.
• Initial dosage for premature atrial and ventricular contractions, paroxysmal AV junctional rhythm, paroxysmal atrial tachycardia, paroxysmal VT, or maintenance after cardioversion of atrial fibrillation or flutter: quinidine sulfate 200 to 400 mg orally every 4 to 6 hours or quinidine gluconate 800 mg added to 40 ml of dextrose 5% in water (D_5W), infused I.V. at 2.5 mg/kg/minute.

What can happen

Adverse cardiovascular effects of quinidine include hypotension, tachycardia, VT, electrocardiogram (ECG) changes (widening of the QRS complex, widened QT and PR intervals), polymorphic VT, AV block, and heart failure.

How you intervene

Keep the following points in mind when caring for a patient taking quinidine:
• Monitor the patient's ECG, heart rate, and blood pressure closely. Don't give more than 4 g/day. Adjust dosages in patients with heart failure and liver disease. (See *Noncardiac adverse effects of quinidine,* page 194.)
• Obtain a baseline QT-interval measurement before the patient begins therapy. Watch for and notify the doctor if the patient develops prolongation of the QT interval, a sign that the patient is predisposed to developing polymorphic VT. Also notify the doctor if the QRS complex widens by 25% or more.
• Remember that quinidine should be avoided in patients with second- or third-degree AV block who don't have pacemakers. It

Noncardiac adverse effects of quinidine

In addition to adverse cardiovascular effects of quinidine, other adverse effects include:
- *CNS:* vertigo, confusion, light-headedness, depression, dementia, headache, tinnitus, hearing loss, visual disturbances
- *Respiratory:* acute asthmatic attack, respiratory arrest
- *GI:* nausea, vomiting, diarrhea, abdominal pain, anorexia, hepatotoxicity
- *Hematologic:* hemolytic anemia, agranulocytosis, fever, thrombocytopenia, anaphylaxis, or allergic reactions including rash
- *Other:* photosensitivity, angioedema.

should also be avoided in patients with profound hypotension, myasthenia gravis, intraventricular conduction defects, or hypersensitivity to the drug. Use it cautiously in elderly patients and in those with renal disease, hepatic disease, or asthma.
- Avoid VT by administering digoxin prior to giving quinidine in patients with atrial tachyarrhythmias.
- Closely monitor patients receiving quinidine and digoxin for signs and symptoms of digoxin toxicity, such as nausea, visual changes, or arrhythmias. Digoxin levels will be increased.
- Ask the patient about herb use. Concomitant use with jimsonweed may adversely affect cardiovascular function. Licorice combined with quinidine use may prolong the patient's QT interval.

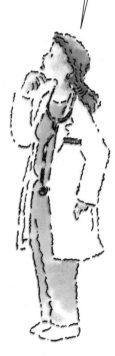

Be alert to the adverse effects of quinidine.

Procainamide hydrochloride

Procainamide hydrochloride (Pronestyl) is indicated for supraventricular and ventricular arrhythmias. Because it comes in a variety of forms, dosages differ.

How to give it

Here's how to administer procainamide:
- Orally: Average dose is 250 to 500 mg every 3 hours; sustained-release (Procan SR), 50 mg/kg daily in divided doses every 6 hours.
- I.M.: Initial daily dose is 50 mg/kg divided into equal doses every 3 to 6 hours.
- I.V.: Slow injection of 50 to 100 mg is given no faster than 25 to 50 mg/minute until one of the following occurs: The arrhythmia is suppressed, the QRS complex widens by 50%, hypotension occurs (often the limiting factor when administering the loading dose), or a total of 500 mg has been given.

Noncardiac adverse effects of procainamide

In addition to adverse cardiovascular effects of procainamide, other dose-related adverse effects include:

- *CNS:* mental depression, hallucinations, seizures, confusion, dizziness
- *GI:* anorexia, nausea, vomiting, abdominal pain, diarrhea, bitter taste, hepatic dysfunction
- *Hematologic:* agranulocytosis, hemolytic anemia, thrombocytopenia, neutropenia
- *Skin:* rash, urticaria
- *Other:* fever, lupus-like syndrome in long-term therapy.

Monitoring procainamide

For patients taking procainamide, you'll need to monitor plasma levels of the drug and its active metabolite *N*-acetylprocainamide (NAPA) to prevent toxic reactions. To suppress ventricular arrhythmias, the therapeutic serum concentration of procainamide should range between 4 and 8 mcg/ml. Therapeutic levels of NAPA should average between 10 and 30 mcg/ml.

- I.V. infusion: 2 g mixed in 500 ml (4 mg/ml) of D_5W and infused at 1 to 4 mg/minute for a maintenance dose.

What can happen

Adverse cardiovascular effects of procainamide include bradycardia, tachycardia, hypotension, worsening heart failure, AV block, polymorphic VT or fibrillation, and asystole.

How you intervene

Keep the following points in mind when caring for a patient taking procainamide:

- Monitor the patient's heart rate, blood pressure, and ECG. Notify the doctor if the patient has hypotension or if you notice widening of the QRS complex by 25% or more. Also report a prolonged QT interval if it's more than half of the R-R interval — a sign that the patient is predisposed to developing polymorphic VT.
- Warn the patient taking procainamide orally not to chew it, which might cause him to get too much of the drug at once. (See *Noncardiac adverse effects of procainamide.*)
- Monitor serum drug levels. (See *Monitoring procainamide.*)
- Remember that procainamide should be avoided in patients with second- or third-degree AV block who don't have pacemakers and in patients with blood dyscrasias, thrombocytopenia, myasthenia gravis, profound hypotension, or known hypersensitivity to the drug. Procainamide may also aggravate digoxin toxicity.

Class Ib antiarrhythmics

Class Ib antiarrhythmics include such drugs as lidocaine (Xylocaine) and tocainide (Tonocard). Because of their actions on the heart, these drugs are effective in suppressing ventricular ectopy but aren't used with supraventricular arrhythmias. (See *Effects of class Ib antiarrhythmics.*) They usually don't have major effects on ECG rhythm.

Lidocaine hydrochloride

Lidocaine was once the drug of choice for suppressing ventricular arrhythmias; however, amiodarone is now favored. When lidocaine is used generally, a patient is first given a loading dose of the drug and then an infusion of it.

How to give it

Here's how to administer lidocaine:
• I.V. bolus injection: 1 to 1.5 mg/kg (usually 50 to 100 mg) at 25 to 50 mg/minute, repeated every 3 to 5 minutes to a maximum of 300 mg total bolus during a 1-hour period.
• I.V. infusion immediately following the bolus dose: 2 g mixed in 500 ml (4 mg/ml) of D_5W and infused at 1 to 4 mg/minute.

What can happen

Cardiovascular adverse effects of lidocaine include AV block, hypotension, bradycardia, new or worsened arrhythmias, and cardiac arrest.

How you intervene

Keep the following points in mind when caring for a patient receiving lidocaine:
• Monitor the patient's heart rate, blood pressure, and ECG.
• Watch for signs and symptoms of drug toxicity. Seizures may be the first sign of toxicity. (See *Noncardiac adverse effects of lidocaine.*) The potential for toxicity is increased if the patient has liver disease, is elderly, is taking cimetidine or propranolol, or receives an infusion of the drug for longer than 24 hours.
• Avoid use of the drug in patients known to be hypersensitive to it or in severe SA, AV, or intraventricular block in the absence of an artificial pacemaker.
• Administer cautiously with other antiarrhythmics.

Tocainide hydrochloride

Tocainide is used to suppress life-threatening ventricular arrhythmias such as sustained VT.

How to give it

The initial dose of tocainide is 400 mg orally every 8 hours. The usual dosage is between 1,200 mg and 1,800 mg daily in three divided doses.

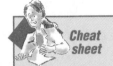

Cheat sheet

Class Ib antiarrhythmics

• Slow phase 0 depolarization
• Don't affect conductivity
• Shorten phase 3 repolarization and action potential

Noncardiac adverse effects of lidocaine

In addition to adverse cardiovascular effects of lidocaine, other adverse effects (mostly dose-related) include:
• *CNS:* seizures, confusion, drowsiness, dizziness, tremors, restlessness, light-headedness, paresthesia, feeling of dissociation, tinnitus, double vision, agitation
• *Respiratory:* respiratory arrest
• *GI:* nausea, vomiting
• *Other:* anaphylaxis.

Effects of class Ib antiarrhythmics

Class Ib antiarrhythmic drugs—such as lidocaine and tocainide—may affect the QRS complexes, as shown on the rhythm strip below. They may also prolong the PR interval. These drugs:

• block sodium influx during phase 0, which depresses the rate of depolarization

• shorten repolarization and the duration of the action potential

• suppress ventricular automaticity in ischemic tissue.

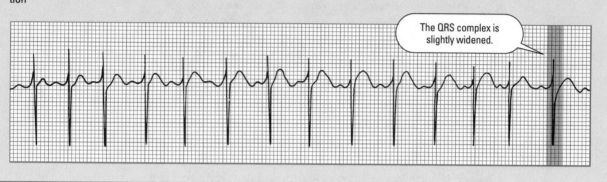

The QRS complex is slightly widened.

What can happen

Adverse cardiovascular effects of tocainide include diaphoresis, bradycardia, hypotension, AV block, palpitations, chest pain, heart failure, and proarrhythmias.

How you intervene

Keep the following points in mind when caring for a patient taking tocainide:
• Monitor the patient's heart rate, blood pressure, and ECG.
• Remember that tocainide should be avoided in patients with second- or third-degree heart block who don't have pacemakers. It should also be avoided in patients with a history of allergic reactions to local amide-type anesthetics.
• Use with caution with other antiarrhythmics, in elderly patients, in heart failure, or in liver or kidney disease.
• Tell the patient to report dyspnea, cough, signs of infection, and bleeding or bruising. These signs and symptoms may indicate a severe adverse reaction to the drug.
• Keep in mind that the risk of toxicity is greater if the patient is receiving cimetidine (Tagamet) at the same time. (See *Noncardiac adverse effects of tocainide*, page 198.)

> ## Noncardiac adverse effects of tocainide
>
> In addition to adverse cardiovascular effects of tocainide, other adverse effects include:
> - *CNS:* mood changes, light-headedness, vertigo, fatigue, tinnitus, headache, dizziness, paresthesia, tremors, confusion, blurred or double vision, seizures, coma
> - *Respiratory:* respiratory arrest, pulmonary fibrosis, pneumonitis, pulmonary edema
> - *GI:* nausea, vomiting, diarrhea, anorexia, abdominal pain
> - *Hematologic:* fever, chills, thrombocytopenia, aplastic anemia, agranulocytosis
> - *Skin:* rash, diaphoresis.

Class Ic antiarrhythmics

Class Ic antiarrhythmic drugs include flecainide (Tambocor) and propafenone (Rythmol). These drugs slow conduction without affecting the duration of the action potential. (See *Effects of class Ic antiarrhythmics.*) Because of their proarrhythmic potential, these drugs are used only for life-threatening or ventricular arrhythmias.

Flecainide acetate

Flecainide is used to treat paroxysmal atrial fibrillation or flutter in patients without structural heart disease and with life-threatening ventricular arrhythmias such as sustained VT. It's also used to prevent paroxysmal supraventricular tachycardia.

How to give it

The dosage for flecainide is 100 to 200 mg orally every 12 hours, to a maximum of 400 mg/day for life-threatening ventricular arrhythmias and 300 mg/day for the prevention of paroxysmal supraventricular tachycardia and paroxysmal atrial fibrillation or flutter in patients without structural heart disease.

What can happen

Adverse cardiovascular effects of flecainide include bradycardia, chest pain, palpitations, heart failure, new or worsened arrhythmias, and cardiac arrest.

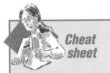

Cheat sheet

Class Ic antiarrhythmics

- Slow conduction
- Don't affect action potential
- Used for life threatening or ventricular arrhythmias

Effects of class Ic antiarrhythmics

Class Ic antiarrhythmic drugs—including flecainide and propafenone—cause the effects shown below on an ECG by exerting particular actions on the cardiac cycle. Class Ic antiarrhythmics block sodium influx during phase 0, which depresses the rate of depolarization. The drugs exert no effect on repolarization or the duration of the action potential.

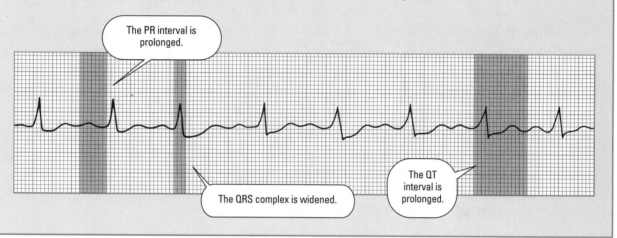

The PR interval is prolonged.

The QRS complex is widened.

The QT interval is prolonged.

How you intervene

Keep the following points in mind when caring for a patient taking flecainide:

• Monitor the patient's heart rate, blood pressure, and ECG. Report widening of the QRS complex by 25% or more, and watch closely for signs of heart failure. (See *Noncardiac adverse effects of flecainide.*)

• Use flecainide cautiously in sick sinus syndrome or in heart, kidney, or liver failure. Avoid its use entirely in second- or third-degree AV block, in bifascicular blocks, and when the patient doesn't have a pacemaker.

Flecainide slows conduction without affecting the action potential.

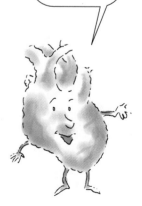

Noncardiac adverse effects of flecainide

In addition to adverse cardiovascular effects of flecainide, other adverse effects include:

• *CNS:* headache, drowsiness, dizziness, syncope, fatigue, blurred vision, tremor, ataxia, vertigo, light-headedness, paresthesia

• *Respiratory:* dyspnea

• *GI:* dry mouth, nausea, vomiting, constipation, abdominal pain, diarrhea.

Noncardiac adverse effects of propafenone

In addition to adverse cardiovascular effects of propafenone, other adverse effects include:
- *CNS:* dizziness, blurred vision, fatigue, headache, paresthesia, anxiety, ataxia, drowsiness, insomnia, syncope, tremors
- *Respiratory:* dyspnea
- *GI:* unusual taste, nausea, vomiting, dyspepsia, constipation, diarrhea, abdominal pain, dry mouth, flatulence
- *Hematologic:* anemia, bruising
- *Other:* joint pain, rash, diaphoresis.

- Administer flecainide cautiously in patients receiving amiodarone, cimetidine, digoxin, or a beta-adrenergic blocker.
- Correct electrolyte imbalances before starting flecainide therapy.

Propafenone hydrochloride

Propafenone slows conduction in all cardiac tissues. The drug is used only for life-threatening ventricular arrhythmias.

How to give it

The usual dosage of propafenone is 150 to 300 mg orally every 8 hours, to a maximum of 900 mg/day.

What can happen

Propafenone's adverse effects on the cardiovascular system include heart failure, AV block, chest pain, bradycardia, atrial fibrillation, bundle-branch block, hypotension, and such proarrhythmias as VT, ventricular fibrillation, and PVCs.

How you intervene

Keep the following points in mind when caring for a patient taking propafenone:
- Monitor the patient's heart rate, blood pressure, and ECG. Report widening of the QRS complex greater than 25%. If widening occurs, the dosage may need to be reduced. Monitor the patient closely for heart failure.
- Remember that propafenone should be avoided in patients with heart failure, cardiogenic shock, sick sinus syndrome without a pacemaker, bronchospastic disorders, hypotension, or SA, AV, or bifascicular blocks.
- Administer propafenone cautiously in patients also receiving cimetidine, other antiarrhythmics such as quinidine, or a beta-

adrenergic blocker. (See *Noncardiac adverse effects of propafenone.*)
• Be aware that patients receiving digoxin along with propafenone might have increased plasma concentration of digoxin, leading to digoxin toxicity.
• Use cautiously in patients also taking an oral anticoagulant because propafenone can increase the plasma concentration of the drug.
• Correct electrolyte imbalances before starting propafenone therapy.
• Instruct the patient to report recurrent or persistent infections.

Class II antiarrhythmics

Class II antiarrhythmic drugs are used to treat supraventricular and ventricular arrhythmias, especially those caused by excess catecholamines. The drugs are called beta-adrenergic blockers because they block beta receptors in the sympathetic nervous system. (See *Effects of class II antiarrhythmics*, page 202.)

Two types of beta receptors exist: beta$_1$ and beta$_2$. Beta$_1$ receptors increase heart rate, contractility, and conductivity. Blocking those receptors decreases the actions listed above.

Beta$_2$ receptors relax smooth muscle in the bronchi and blood vessels. Keep in mind that blocking these receptors may result in vasoconstriction and bronchospasm.

Beta-adrenergic blockers that block only beta$_1$ receptors are referred to as cardioselective. Those that block both beta$_1$ and beta$_2$ receptors are referred to as noncardioselective.

Beta-adrenergic blockers

The following beta-adrenergic blockers are Food and Drug Administration–approved for use as antiarrhythmics:
• acebutolol (Sectral). This drug is classified as cardioselective. It decreases contractility and heart rate. The normal dosage is 200 mg orally twice daily, increased as needed to a usual dosage of 600 to 1,200 mg daily.
• propranolol (Inderal). This drug is classified as noncardioselective. It decreases heart rate and contractility. Propranolol reduces the incidence of sudden cardiac death after myocardial infarction (MI). It may be given orally or I.V. The oral dosage is 10 to 30 mg three or four times daily. The I.V. dosage is 0.5 to 3 mg, at a rate not to exceed 1 mg/minute. After 3 mg have been given, another dose may be given in 2 minutes; subsequent doses may be given no sooner then every 4 hours.

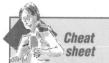

Cheat sheet

Class II antiarrhythmics

• *acebutolol (Sectral):* decreases contractility and heart rate
• *propranolol:* decreases heart rate and contractility
• *esmolol:* decreases heart rate, contractility, and blood pressure
• *sotalol:* decreases heart rate and cardiac output, slows AV conduction, and lowers systolic and diastolic blood pressure
• Avoid in patients with bradycardia, second- or third-degree AV block, and shock

Effects of class II antiarrhythmics

Class II antiarrhythmic drugs—including such beta-adrenergic blockers as propranolol, esmolol, acebutolol, and sotalol—cause certain effects on an ECG (as shown here) by exerting particular actions on the cardiac cycle. Class II antiarrhythmics:

- depress SA node automaticity
- shorten the duration of the action potential
- increase the refractory period of atrial and AV junctional tissues, which slows conduction
- inhibit sympathetic activity.

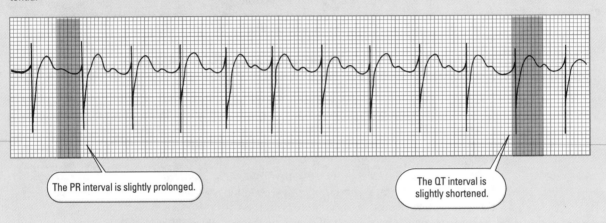

The PR interval is slightly prolonged.

The QT interval is slightly shortened.

- esmolol (Brevibloc). This drug is a short-acting cardioselective drug that decreases heart rate, contractility, and blood pressure administered by I.V. titration. The loading dose is 500 mcg/kg over 1 minute, then 50 mcg/kg/minute for 4 minutes, titrated until the desired effect is achieved. Maximum maintenance dose is 200 mcg/kg/minute
- sotalol (Betapace). This drug is a noncardioselective drug that also has class III characteristics. It decreases heart rate, slows AV conduction, decreases cardiac output, and lowers systolic and diastolic blood pressure. The initial dosage is 80 mg orally twice daily. Most patients respond to a daily dose of 160 to 320 mg.

What can happen

The adverse effects of beta-adrenergic blockers on the cardiovascular system may vary, but they include bradycardia, hypotension, AV block, heart failure, chest pain, and palpitations.

How you intervene

Keep the following points in mind when caring for a patient taking a beta-adrenergic blocker:
- Monitor the patient's heart rate, blood pressure, and ECG.

Class II anti-arrhythmic drugs act on the cardiac cycle.

Noncardiac adverse effects of class II beta-adrenergic blockers

In addition to adverse cardiovascular effects of class II beta-adrenergic blockers, other adverse effects include:
• *CNS:* insomnia, syncope, mental depression, emotional ability, fatigue, headache, dizziness, lethargy, vivid dreams, hallucinations, light-headedness
• *Respiratory:* dyspnea, bronchospasm, especially in patients with asthma or other bronchospastic disease
• *Hematologic:* thrombocytopenia, agranulocytosis, alterations in blood sugar level
• *Skin:* rash.

• Remember that beta-adrenergic blockers should be avoided in patients with bradycardia, second- or third-degree AV block, and shock. Use them cautiously in patients with diabetes mellitus (they mask the signs of hypoglycemia), heart failure, kidney disease, hyperthyroidism, liver disease, myasthenia gravis, peripheral vascular disease, and hypotension.
• Keep in mind that noncardioselective beta-adrenergic blockers are contraindicated in patients with asthma or other bronchospastic disease. (See *Noncardiac adverse effects of class II beta-adrenergic blockers.*)
• Remember that beta-adrenergic blockers diminish the patient's ability to withstand exercise because the heart rate can't increase. These drugs also block sympathetic response to shock.
• Correct electrolyte imbalances before starting therapy with a beta blocker.

Class III antiarrhythmics

Class III antiarrhythmics are called potassium channel blockers. (See *Effects of class III antiarrhythmics,* page 204.) They include amiodarone (Cordarone) and ibutilide fumarate (Corvert). Sotalol has qualities of both class II and class III antiarrhythmics. All class III antiarrhythmics have prearrhythmic potential.

Amiodarone

Amiodarone is used to treat supraventricular arrhythmias, paroxysmal supraventricular tachycardia caused by ventricular arrhythmias, and accessory pathway conduction such as Wolff-Parkinson-

Effects of class III antiarrhythmics

Class III antiarrhythmic drugs—including amiodarone, sotalol, and ibutilide—cause the effects shown below on an ECG by exerting particular actions on the cardiac cycle. Class III antiarrhythmics:

- block potassium movement during phase 3
- increase the duration of the action potential
- prolong the effective refractory period.

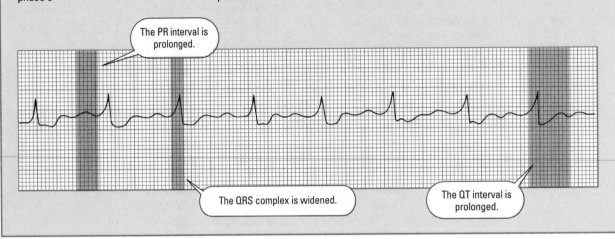

The PR interval is prolonged.

The QRS complex is widened.

The QT interval is prolonged.

White syndrome. Use of amiodarone is limited because of its adverse effects. (See *Noncardiac adverse effects of amiodarone.*)

Take care not to confuse amiodarone with amrinone (Inocor), which is a positive inotropic agent.

How to give it

Here's how to administer amiodarone:
- Orally: 800 to 1,600 mg daily in divided doses for 1 to 3 weeks, followed by 600 to 800 mg/day for 4 weeks, followed by 200 to 600 mg/day as a maintenance dosage.
- I.V. infusion: 150 mg mixed in 100 ml D_5W and infused over 10 minutes (15 mg/minute); then 900 mg mixed in 500 ml D_5W with 360 mg infused over the next 6 hours (1 mg/minute); followed by 540 mg infused over 18 hours (0.5 mg/minute). After the first 24 hours, a maintenance I.V. infusion of 720 mg/24 hours (0.5 mg/minute) should be continued.

What can happen

Adverse effects of amiodarone given by I.V. infusion include bradycardia, hypotension, VT, AV block, cardiogenic shock, heart failure, asystole, and pulseless electrical activity.

Long-term oral therapy is associated with bradycardia, sinus arrest, SA block, AV block, and hypotension.

Noncardiac adverse effects of amiodarone

In addition to adverse cardiovascular effects of amiodarone, other adverse effects include:
• *CNS:* malaise, fatigue, dizziness, peripheral neuropathy, ataxia, paresthesia, tremors, headache, visual disturbances
• *Respiratory:* pulmonary toxicity (progressive dyspnea, cough, fever, pleuritic chest pain)
• *GI:* nausea, vomiting, constipation, anorexia, abdominal pain
• *Other:* photosensitivity, abnormal taste and smell, hypothyroidism or hyperthyroidism, bleeding disorders.

How you intervene

Keep the following points in mind when caring for a patient taking amiodarone:
• Monitor the patient's vital signs, ECG, and respiratory status.
• Monitor laboratory test results, such as electrolyte levels, liver function studies, thyroid function studies, pulmonary function studies, and chest X-rays.
• Check for signs of digoxin toxicity or increased prothrombin time. Amiodarone can increase the serum levels of digoxin and oral anticoagulants.
• Remember that amiodarone should be avoided in patients with hypersensitivity to the drug, cardiogenic shock, marked sinus bradycardia, and second- or third-degree AV block without a pacemaker. Use the drug cautiously in patients with cardiomegaly, pre-existing bradycardia or sinus node disease, conduction disturbances, or depressed ventricular function.
• Be aware that the drug has a long half-life (56 days) and therefore takes a long time for the drug to reach therapeutic levels and to be cleared by the body.
• Know that amiodarone may increase theophylline levels in patients taking theophylline. Monitor the patient for signs of theophylline toxicity.
• Be aware that amiodarone may decrease phenytoin levels. Monitor phenytoin levels closely.
• Instruct the patient to wear sunscreen and protective clothing to avoid photosensitivity reactions. A blue-gray discoloration of exposed skin may occur.
• Recommend that the patient have yearly ophthalmic examinations. Within 1 to 4 months after beginning amiodarone

Tell the patient taking amiodarone to wear sunscreen and protective clothing to avoid photosensitivity reactions.

therapy, most patients show corneal microdeposits upon slit-lamp ophthalmic examination. Instillation of methylcellulose ophthalmic solution minimizes corneal microdeposits.
• Administer the drug through a central venous catheter to avoid phlebitis.

Ibutilide fumarate

Ibutilide fumarate is becoming increasingly popular for the rapid conversion of recent-onset atrial fibrillation or flutter to sinus rhythm. The drug increases atrial and ventricular refractoriness.

How to give it

If your adult patient weighs 132 lb (60 kg) or more, he'll receive 1 mg of ibutilide fumarate I.V. over 10 minutes. If he weighs less than 132 lb, the dose is 0.01 mg/kg.

Ibutilide fumarate may be diluted in 50 ml of normal saline solution or D_5W. Should the arrhythmia still be present 10 minutes after the infusion is complete, the dose may be repeated.

What can happen

Adverse cardiovascular effects of ibutilide fumarate include PVCs, VT, sustained polymorphic VT, hypotension, bundle-branch block, AV block, hypertension, bradycardia, tachycardia, palpitations, and lengthening of the QT interval. Noncardiac adverse effects include headache and nausea.

How you intervene

Keep these points in mind when giving ibutilide fumarate:
• Monitor the patient's vital signs and ECG continuously during the infusion and for at least 4 hours afterward. The infusion will be stopped if the arrhythmia terminates or if the patient develops VT or marked prolongation of the QT interval, which signals the possible development of polymorphic VT.
• Have emergency equipment and medication nearby for the treatment of sustained VT.
• Ibutilide fumarate isn't recommended for patients with a history of polymorphic VT.
• The drug should be used cautiously in patients receiving digoxin (Lanoxin) because it can mask signs and symptoms of cardiotoxicity associated with excessive digoxin levels.
• Don't administer ibutilide fumarate at the same time or within 4 hours of class Ia or other class III antiarrhythmics.
• Don't give ibutilide fumarate with other drugs that prolong the QT interval, such as phenothiazines and tricyclic or tetracyclic antidepressants.

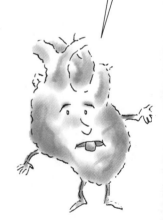

Adverse effects of ibutilide include PVCs, VT, hypotension (gulp), AV block (gulp)... Is it getting hot in here?

• Patients with atrial fibrillation that has lasted more than 2 days must receive anticoagulants for at least 2 weeks prior to the initiation of ibutilide therapy.

Class IV antiarrhythmics

Class IV antiarrhythmic drugs are called calcium channel blockers. They include verapamil (Calan) and diltiazem (Cardizem). These drugs prolong conduction time and the refractory period in the AV node. (See *Effects of class IV antiarrhythmics.*)

Other calcium channel blockers, including nifedipine (Procardia), don't cause electrophysiologic changes and aren't used as antiarrhythmics. They're used primarily to treat hypertension.

Verapamil hydrochloride

Verapamil is used for paroxysmal supraventricular tachycardia because of its effect on the AV node. It also slows the ventricular response in atrial fibrillation and flutter.

How to give it

Here's how to administer verapamil:
• Orally for chronic atrial fibrillation: 80 to 120 mg three or four times a day to a maximum of 480 mg/day.

Effects of class IV antiarrhythmics

Class IV antiarrhythmic drugs—including such calcium channel blockers as verapamil and diltiazem—affect the cardiac cycle in specific ways and may lead to the ECG change shown here. Class IV antiarrhythmics:

• block calcium movement during phase 2

• prolong the conduction time and increase the refractory period in the AV node

• decrease contractility.

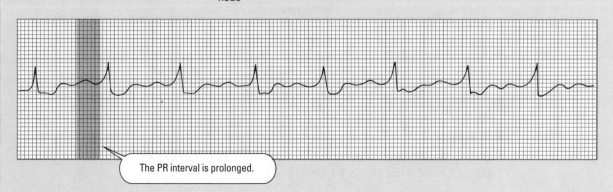

The PR interval is prolonged.

Noncardiac adverse effects of verapamil

In addition to adverse cardiovascular effects of verapamil, other adverse effects include:

- *CNS:* headache, dizziness
- *Respiratory:* dyspnea
- *GI:* nausea, constipation, elevated liver enzymes
- *Skin:* rash.

- I.V. injection for supraventricular arrhythmias: 0.075 to 0.15 mg/kg (usually 5 to 10 mg) over 2 minutes; may repeat in 30 minutes if no response occurs.

What can happen

Cardiovascular adverse effects of verapamil include bradycardia or tachycardia, AV block, hypotension, heart failure, edema, flushing, and ventricular fibrillation.

How you intervene

Keep the following points in mind when caring for a patient taking verapamil:

- Monitor the patient's heart rate, blood pressure, and ECG. Also monitor liver function studies. (See *Noncardiac adverse effects of verapamil.*)
- Note that calcium may be given before verapamil to prevent hypotension.
- Advise the patient to change position slowly to avoid orthostatic hypotension.
- Remember that verapamil should be avoided in sick sinus syndrome or second- or third-degree AV block without a pacemaker and in atrial fibrillation or flutter due to Wolff-Parkinson-White syndrome. It also should be avoided in patients with hypersensitivity to the drug, advanced heart failure, cardiogenic shock, profound hypotension, acute MI, or pulmonary edema.
- Give the drug cautiously to patients receiving digoxin or oral beta-adrenergic blockers, elderly patients, and patients with heart failure, hypotension, liver disease, and kidney disease. Don't give verapamil to patients receiving I.V. beta-adrenergic blockers.

Diltiazem

Diltiazem is administered I.V. to treat paroxysmal supraventricular tachycardia and atrial fibrillation or flutter. Diltiazem is also used

> ### Noncardiac adverse effects of diltiazem
>
> In addition to adverse cardiovascular effects of diltiazem, other adverse effects include:
> - *CNS:* headache, drowsiness, dizziness, weakness
> - *GI:* nausea, transient elevation of liver enzymes, constipation, abdominal discomfort, acute hepatic injury
> - *Skin:* rash.

to treat angina and hypertension, but those uses aren't discussed here.

How to give it

Here's how to give diltiazem:
- I.V. injection: 0.25 mg/kg (usually 20 mg) over 2 minutes; may repeat in 15 minutes at 0.35 mg/kg (usually 25 mg) over 2 minutes.
- I.V. infusion: 125 mg mixed in 100 ml normal saline solution or D_5W for a total volume of 125 ml (1 mg/ml) of solution and infused at a rate of 5 to 15 mg/hour (usually 10 mg/hour).

What can happen

Adverse cardiovascular effects of diltiazem include edema, flushing, bradycardia, hypotension, heart failure, arrhythmias, conduction abnormalities, sinus node dysfunction, and AV block.

How you intervene

Keep the following points in mind when caring for a patient receiving diltiazem:
- Monitor the patient's heart rate, blood pressure, and ECG.
- Diltiazem should be avoided in patients with sick sinus syndrome or second- or third-degree AV block without a pacemaker, atrial fibrillation or flutter due to Wolff-Parkinson-White syndrome, advanced heart failure, cardiogenic shock, profound hypotension, acute MI, pulmonary edema, or sensitivity to the drug.
- Use cautiously in elderly patients; in patients with heart failure, hypotension, or liver or kidney disease; and in those receiving digoxin or beta-adrenergic blockers. (See *Noncardiac adverse effects of diltiazem.*)
- Don't give to patients receiving I.V. beta-adrenergic blockers.

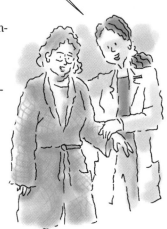

Use diltiazem cautiously in elderly patients.

• Advise the patient to change position slowly to avoid postural hypotension.

Unclassified antiarrhythmics

Some antiarrhythmic drugs defy categorization. Let's look at some of those drugs, which are called unclassified or miscellaneous antiarrhythmic drugs.

Adenosine

Adenosine is a naturally occurring nucleoside used to treat paroxysmal supraventricular tachycardia. It acts on the AV node to slow conduction and inhibit reentry pathways. It's also useful in treating paroxysmal supraventricular tachycardia associated with Wolff-Parkinson-White syndrome.

Although adenosine isn't effective for atrial fibrillation or atrial flutter, it does slow the rate in paroxysmal supraventricular tachycardia enough to determine the rhythm so that a more appropriate agent such as verapamil can be used.

How to give it

Administer 6 mg of adenosine I.V. over 1 to 2 seconds, immediately followed by a rapid flush with 20 ml of normal saline solution. Because the drug's half-life is less than 10 seconds, it needs to reach the circulation quickly. Repeat with an injection of 12 mg of adenosine if the rhythm doesn't convert within 1 to 2 minutes.

What can happen

Adverse cardiovascular effects of adenosine include transient arrhythmias such as a short asystolic pause at the time of conversion. Other adverse effects include hypotension (if large doses are used), facial flushing, diaphoresis, chest pressure, and recurrence of the arrhythmia. (See *Noncardiac adverse effects of adenosine.*)

Noncardiac adverse effects of adenosine

In addition to adverse cardiovascular effects of adenosine, other adverse effects include:
• *CNS:* apprehension, light-headedness, burning sensation, headache, numbness and tingling in arms
• *Respiratory:* dyspnea
• *GI:* nausea.

How you intervene

Keep the following points in mind when caring for a patient receiving adenosine:
• Monitor the patient's heart rate, blood pressure, ECG, ventilatory rate and depth, and breath sounds for wheezes.
• Remember that adenosine should be avoided in patients with hypersensitivity to the drug, second- or third-degree AV block, or sick sinus syndrome without a pacemaker. Use cautiously in older adults and in patients with asthma or those receiving dipyridamole (Persantine) or carbamazepine (Tegretol).
• Store adenosine at room temperature.
• The patient may require a higher dose or not respond to therapy at all if he's also taking aminophylline or another xanthine derivative.

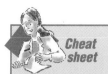

Cheat sheet

Atropine use

• Atropine: anticholinergic drug
• Blocks vagal effects on the SA and AV nodes
• Speeds heart rate
• Enhances conduction through the AV node

Atropine

Atropine is an anticholinergic drug that blocks vagal effects on the SA and AV nodes. This enhances conduction through the AV node and speeds the heart rate. Atropine is used to treat symptomatic bradycardia and asystole. However, atropine is ineffective in patients following dissection of the vagus nerve during heart transplant surgery. Isoproterenol (Isuprel) can be used to treat symptomatic bradycardia in these patients.

How to give it

Administer atropine by a 0.5- to 1-mg I.V. injection repeated as needed at 3- to 5-minute intervals, to a maximum dose of 0.04 mg/kg. The initial dose for asystole is 1 mg. The maximum dose is 3 mg.

What can happen

Adverse cardiovascular effects of atropine include tachycardia (with high doses), palpitations, bradycardia if given slowly or in a dose of less than 0.5 mg, hypotension, and chest pain and in-

Noncardiac adverse effects of atropine

Noncardiac adverse effects of atropine include:
• *CNS:* ataxia, disorientation, delirium, agitation, confusion, headache, restlessness, insomnia, dizziness, blurred vision, dilated pupils, photophobia
• *GI:* dry mouth, constipation, paralytic ileus, nausea, and vomiting
• *GU:* urine retention
• *Other:* increased intraocular pressure anaphylaxis, urticaria.

creased myocardial oxygen consumption in patients with coronary artery disease.

How you intervene

Keep the following points in mind when caring for a patient receiving atropine:
• Monitor the patient's heart rate, blood pressure, ECG, urine output, and bowel sounds. (See *Noncardiac adverse effects of atropine*, page 211.)
• Remember that atropine should be avoided in patients with hypersensitivity to belladonna, acute angle-closure glaucoma, GI obstruction, obstructive uropathy, myasthenia gravis, and tachyarrhythmias.
• Use atropine cautiously in patients with renal disease, heart failure, hyperthyroidism, hepatic disease, hypertension, and acute MI. Don't give atropine for bradycardia unless the patient is symptomatic. Increasing the heart rate in these patients can lead to increased myocardial oxygen consumption and a worsening of the infarction.

Digoxin

Digoxin (Lanoxin) is used to treat paroxysmal supraventricular tachycardia and atrial fibrillation and flutter, especially in patients with heart failure. It provides antiarrhythmic effects by enhancing vagal tone and slowing conduction through the SA and AV nodes. It also strengthens myocardial contraction. Digoxin has visible effects on the patient's ECG. (See *Digoxin: ECG effects.*)

How to give it

To administer digoxin rapidly and orally or I.V., give a digitalizing dose of 0.5 to 1 mg divided into two or more doses every 6 to 8 hours. The usual maintenance dosage is 0.125 to 0.5 mg daily.

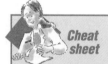

Cheat sheet

Digoxin use

• Use to treat paroxysmal supraventricular tachycardia and atrial fibrillation and flutter, especially in patients with heart failure.
• Cardiac effects of digoxin toxicity include SA and AV blocks and junctional and ventricular arrhythmias.
• Avoid in patients with known hypersensitivity to the drug, sick sinus syndrome, SA or AV block, ventricular tachycardia, hypertrophic cardiomyopathy, or Wolff-Parkinson-White syndrome.

Noncardiac adverse effects of digoxin

In addition to adverse cardiovascular effects of digoxin, other adverse effects resulting from toxicity include:
• *CNS:* headache, visual disturbances, hallucinations, fatigue, muscle weakness, agitation, malaise, dizziness, stupor, paresthesia
• *GI:* anorexia, nausea, vomiting, diarrhea
• *Other:* yellow-green halos around visual images, blurred vision, light flashes, photophobia, and diplopia.

Digoxin: ECG effects

Digoxin affects the cardiac cycle in various ways and may lead to the ECG changes shown here.

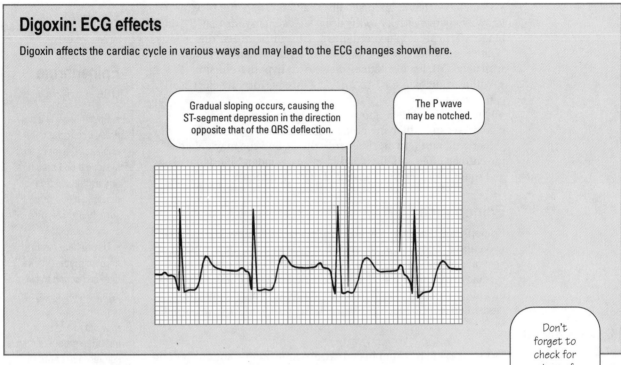

Gradual sloping occurs, causing the ST-segment depression in the direction opposite that of the QRS deflection.

The P wave may be notched.

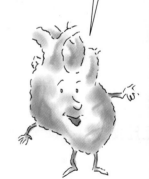

Don't forget to check for signs of digoxin toxicity.

What can happen

Too much digoxin in the body causes toxicity. Toxic cardiac effects include SA and AV blocks and junctional and ventricular arrhythmias. Digoxin toxicity is treated by discontinuing digoxin; correcting oxygenation and electrolyte imbalances; treating arrhythmias with phenytoin, lidocaine, atropine, or a pacemaker; giving digoxin immune fab (Digibind) to reverse life-threatening arrhythmias or blocks (occurs within 30 to 60 minutes); and correcting the potassium level before giving digoxin immune fab.

How you intervene

Keep the following points in mind when caring for a patient receiving digoxin:
• Check for signs of digoxin toxicity, especially in patients with hypokalemia, hypocalcemia, hypercalcemia, or hypomagnesemia. Monitor serum electrolyte levels as ordered.
• Monitor the patient's apical heart rate and ECG. A heart rate below 60 beats/minute or a change in rhythm can signal digoxin toxicity. If this occurs, withhold digoxin and notify the doctor. (See *Noncardiac adverse effects of digoxin.*)

• Remember that digoxin should be avoided in patients with known hypersensitivity to the drug, sick sinus syndrome, SA or AV block, VT, hypertrophic cardiomyopathy, or Wolff-Parkinson-White syndrome. Use cautiously in older adults and in patients with acute MI, liver or kidney disease, or hypothyroidism.
• Withhold digoxin for 1 to 2 days before performing electrical cardioversion.
• Question the patient about herbal preparation use because digoxin reacts with many preparations. Fumitory, lily of the valley, goldenseal, motherwort, Shepard's purse, and rue may enhance the cardiac effects of digoxin. Licorice, oleander, Siberian ginseng, and squill may increase the risk of digoxin toxicity.

Epinephrine

Epinephrine is a naturally occurring catecholamine. It acts directly on alpha- and beta-adrenergic receptor sites of the sympathetic nervous system, and it's used to help restore cardiac rhythm in cardiac arrest and to treat symptomatic bradycardia. Its actions include increasing the systolic blood pressure and slightly decreasing diastolic blood pressure, heart rate, and cardiac output.

How to give it

To restore sinus rhythm in cardiac arrest in adults, administer epinephrine by I.V. injection as a 1-mg dose (10 ml of 1:10,000 solution). Each dose given by peripheral injection should be followed by a 20-ml flush of I.V. fluid to ensure quick delivery of the drug. Doses may be repeated every 3 to 5 minutes as needed. (Some clinicians advocate doses of up to 5 mg, especially for patients who don't respond to the usual I.V. dose.) After initial I.V. administration, an infusion may be given at 1 to 4 mcg/minute.

What can happen

Adverse cardiovascular effects include palpitations, hypertension, tachycardia, ventricular fibrillation, anginal pain, shock, and ECG changes, including a decreased T-wave amplitude.

How you intervene

Keep these points in mind when administering epinephrine:
• Be sure to note the concentration of the epinephrine solution used. (Remember that 1 mg equals 1 ml of 1:1,000 or 10 ml of 1:10,000 concentration.)
• When administering I.V. epinephrine, monitor the patient's heart rate, ECG rhythm, and blood pressure throughout therapy. (See *Noncardiac adverse effects of epinephrine*.)

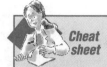

Cheat sheet

Epinephrine use

• Epinephrine is a naturally occurring catecholamine; it increases systolic blood pressure and slightly decreases diastolic blood pressure, heart rate, and cardiac output.
• Use to help restore cardiac rhythm in cardiac arrest and to treat symptomatic bradycardia.
• Avoid use of epinephrine products with sulfites in patients with sulfite allergies, except in the case of emergency.

Noncardiac adverse effects of epinephrine

In addition to adverse cardiovascular effects of epinephrine, other adverse effects include:
- *CNS:* nervousness, tremor, dizziness, vertigo, headache, disorientation, agitation, fear, pallor, weakness, cerebral hemorrhage and, in patients with Parkinson's disease, increased rigidity and tremor
- *Respiratory:* dyspnea
- *GI:* nausea, vomiting
- *Other:* tissue necrosis.

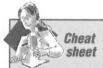

Cheat sheet

Magnesium sulfate use

- Use to treat ventricular arrhythmias, especially polymorphic ventricular tachycardia.
- Avoid in patients with renal disease.
- Have I.V. calcium available to counteract effects of hypermagnesemia.

- Don't mix the drug with alkaline solutions. Use D$_5$W, lactated Ringer's solution, or normal saline solution or a combination of dextrose and saline solution.
- Some epinephrine products contain sulfites. Use of those products normally should be avoided in patient's with sulfite allergies. The only exception is when epinephrine is being used in an emergency.
- Remember that the use of epinephrine with digoxin (Lanoxin) or such general anesthetics as cyclopropane or a halogenated hydrocarbon like halothane (Fluothane) may increase the risk of ventricular arrhythmias.
- Avoid giving epinephrine with other drugs that exert a similar effect. Doing so can cause severe adverse cardiovascular effects.

Magnesium sulfate

Magnesium sulfate is used to treat ventricular arrhythmias, especially polymorphic VT and paroxysmal atrial tachycardia. It's also used as a preventive measure in acute MI. Magnesium sulfate acts similarly to class III antiarrhythmic drugs because it decreases myocardial cell excitability and conduction. It slows conduction through the AV node and prolongs the refractory period in the atria and ventricles.

How to give it

For life-threatening arrhythmias, administer 1 to 2 g magnesium sulfate mixed in 50 to 100 ml of D$_5$W administered over 5 to 60 minutes. Follow with an infusion of 0.5 to 1 g/hour. The dosage and duration of therapy depend on the patient's response and serum magnesium levels. The optimum dosage is still under study.

> ## Noncardiac adverse effects of magnesium sulfate
>
> In addition to adverse cardiovascular effects of magnesium sulfate, other adverse effects include:
> - *CNS:* drowsiness, depressed reflexes, flaccid paralysis, hypothermia
> - *Respiratory:* respiratory paralysis
> - *Other:* hypocalcemia.

What can happen

Adverse cardiovascular effects of magnesium sulfate include diaphoresis, flushing, depressed cardiac function, bradycardia, hypotension, and circulatory collapse.

How you intervene

Keep the following points in mind when caring for a patient receiving magnesium sulfate:
- Monitor the patient's heart rate, blood pressure, ventilatory rate, ECG, urine output, deep tendon reflexes, and mental status. (See *Noncardiac adverse effects of magnesium sulfate.*)
- Remember that magnesium sulfate should be avoided in patients with renal disease. Use it cautiously in patients with renal insufficiency and in those taking digoxin.
- Monitor closely for signs and symptoms of hypermagnesemia, such as hypotension, AV block, central nervous system depression, depressed or absent deep tendon reflexes, muscle weakness or paralysis, and respiratory arrest.
- Have I.V. calcium available to counteract the effects of hypermagnesemia.
- Have intubation equipment and a mechanical ventilator available.
- Magnesium sulfate is contraindicated in heart block and in patients with myocardial damage.

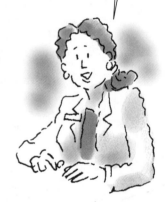

Avoid magnesium sulfate in patients with renal disease.

Teaching about antiarrhythmics

Here are some important points to emphasize when teaching your patient about antiarrhythmic drugs:
- Take the drug exactly as prescribed. Don't stop taking the drugs without consulting your doctor.

• Call the doctor if the following occur: chest pain, shortness of breath, cough, palpitations, dizziness, fatigue, a weight gain of more than 2 lb (0.9 kg) per day, a very fast or slow heart rate, a change in the regularity of the heartbeat, or persistent changes you feel might be related to drug therapy.
• See your doctor for regular checkups, as scheduled. Periodic physical examinations, ECGs, chest X-rays, and laboratory studies will help evaluate the effectiveness of therapy.
• Use herbal preparations with care. Some can cause life-threatening interactions.

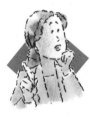

Quick quiz

1. Antiarrhythmic drugs that depress the rate of depolarization belong to class:
  A.   I.
  B.   II.
  C.   III.
Answer: A. Class I antiarrhythmic drugs block sodium influx during phase 0, depressing the rate of depolarization.

2. The antiarrhythmic drug used to treat PVCs or ventricular arrhythmias that should be administered by slow I.V. injection (no faster than 25 to 50 mcg/minute every 5 minutes) is:
  A.   atropine.
  B.   procainamide.
  C.   magnesium sulfate.
Answer: B. Procainamide should be administered by slow I.V. injection (25 to 50 mcg/minute every 5 minutes) until the arrhythmia is suppressed, the QRS complex widens by 50%, hypotension occurs, or a total of 1 g has been given.

3. The drug that blocks vagal stimulation and increases the heart rate is:
  A.   atropine.
  B.   diltiazem.
  C.   verapamil.
Answer: A. Atropine blocks vagal effects on the SA node, enhances conduction through the node, and speeds the heart rate. The drug is used to treat symptomatic bradycardia.

4.   The class II antiarrhythmic drug used for the rapid conversion of recent onset atrial fibrillation or flutter to sinus rhythm is:

    A.   digoxin.
    B.   ibutilide fumarate.
    C.   procainamide.

Answer: B. Ibutilide fumarate increases atrial and ventricular refractoriness and is used for the rapid conversion of recent onset atrial fibrillation or flutter.

5.   The drugs known for lowering the resting heart rate are:

    A.   beta-adrenergic blockers.
    B.   potassium channel blockers.
    C.   sodium channel blockers.

Answer: A. Beta-adrenergic blockers block sympathetic nervous system beta receptors and lower heart rate, contractility, and conduction.

Scoring

☆☆☆   If you answered all five questions correctly, just say wow! You're the antiarrhythmic drug czar!

☆☆   If you answered three or four questions correctly, great job! You're the deputy antiarrhythmic drug czar!

☆   If you answered fewer than three questions correctly, no worries. You're the antiarrhythmic drug czar's sergeant at arms!

Part IV

The 12-lead ECG

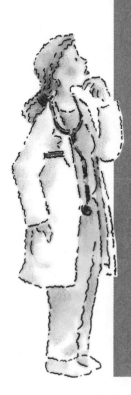

11

Obtaining a 12-lead ECG

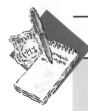

Just the facts

This chapter focuses on the 12-lead ECG, which gives a more complete view of the heart's electrical activity than a rhythm strip. In this chapter, you'll learn:

♦ how the 12-lead ECG helps diagnose pathologic conditions

♦ how the heart's electrical axis relates to the 12-lead ECG

♦ how to prepare your patient, place the electrodes, and record the ECG

♦ the diagnostic purposes of the posterior-lead ECG and the right chest lead ECG

♦ the function of a signal-averaged ECG.

A look at the 12-lead ECG

The 12-lead ECG is a diagnostic test that helps identify pathologic conditions, especially angina and acute myocardial infarction (MI). It gives a more complete view of the heart's electrical activity than a rhythm strip and can be used to assess left ventricular function. Patients with other conditions that affect the heart's electrical system may also benefit from a 12-lead ECG. (See *Why a 12-lead ECG?*)

Interdependent evidence

Like other diagnostic tests, a 12-lead ECG must be viewed alongside other clinical evidence. Always correlate the patient's ECG results with his history, physical assessment findings, laboratory results, and medication regimen.

Remember, too, that an ECG can be done in a variety of ways, including over a telephone line. (See *Transtelephonic cardiac monitoring*, page 223.) Transtelephonic monitoring, in fact, has

Why a 12-lead ECG?

A 12-lead ECG is usually performed on patients having a myocardial infarction. In addition, this diagnostic test may be ordered for patients with other conditions that also affect the heart, including:

• arrhythmia
• heart chamber enlargement
• digoxin or other drug toxicity
• electrolyte imbalance
• pulmonary embolism
• pericarditis
• hypothermia.

become increasingly important as a tool for assessing patients at home and in other nonclinical settings.

How leads work

The 12-lead ECG records the heart's electrical activity using a series of electrodes placed on the patient's extremities and chest wall. The 12 leads include three bipolar limb leads (I, II, and III), three unipolar augmented limb leads (aV_R, aV_L, and aV_F), and six unipolar precordial, or chest, leads (V_1, V_2, V_3, V_4, V_5, and V_6). These leads provide 12 different views of the heart's electrical activity. (See *A look at the leads*, page 224.)

Up, down, and across

Scanning up, down, and across the heart, each lead transmits information about a different area. The waveforms obtained from each lead vary depending on the location of the lead in relation to the wave of depolarization, or electrical stimulus, passing through the myocardium.

Limb leads

The six limb leads record electrical activity in the heart's frontal plane. This plane is a view through the middle of the heart from top to bottom. Electrical activity is recorded from the anterior to the posterior axis.

Precordial leads

The six precordial leads provide information on electrical activity in the heart's horizontal plane, a transverse view through the middle of the heart, dividing it into upper and lower portions. Electrical activity is recorded from either a superior or an inferior approach.

The electrical axis

Besides assessing 12 different leads, a 12-lead ECG records the heart's electrical axis. The axis is a measurement of electrical impulses flowing through the heart.

As impulses travel through the heart, they generate small electrical forces called instantaneous vectors. The mean of these vectors represents the force and direction of the wave of depolarization through the heart. That mean is called the electrical axis. It's also called the mean instantaneous vector and the mean QRS vector.

Transtelephonic cardiac monitoring

Using a special recorder-transmitter, patients at home can transmit ECGs by telephone to a central monitoring center for immediate interpretation. This technique, called transtelephonic cardiac monitoring (TTM), reduces health care costs and is widely used.

Nurses play an important role in TTM. Besides performing extensive patient and family teaching, they may run the central monitoring center and help interpret ECGs sent by patients.

TTM allows the health care professional to assess transient conditions that cause such symptoms as palpitations, dizziness, syncope, confusion, paroxysmal dyspnea, and chest pain. Such conditions, which commonly don't show themselves while the patient is in the presence of a health care professional, can make diagnosis difficult and costly.

With TTM, the patient can transmit an ECG recording from his home when the symptoms appear, avoiding the need to go to the hospital for diagnosis and offering a greater opportunity for early diagnosis. Even if symptoms don't appear often, the patient can keep the equipment for long periods of time, which further aids in the diagnosis of the patient's condition.

Home care

TTM can also be used by patients having cardiac rehabilitation at home. You'll call the patient regularly during this period to receive transmissions and assess progress. Because of this continuous monitoring, TTM can help reduce the anxiety felt by many patients and their families after discharge, especially if the patient suffered a myocardial infarction.

TTM is especially valuable for assessing the effects of drugs and for diagnosing and managing paroxysmal arrhythmias. In both cases, TTM can eliminate the need for admitting the patient for evaluation and a potentially lengthy hospital stay.

Understanding TTM equipment

TTM requires three main pieces of equipment: an ECG recorder-transmitter, a standard telephone line, and a receiver. The ECG recorder-transmitter converts electrical activity picked up from the patient's heart into acoustic waves. Some models contain built-in memory that stores a recording of the activity so the patient can transmit it later.

A standard telephone line is used to transmit information. The receiver converts the acoustic waves transmitted over the telephone line into ECG activity, which is then recorded on ECG paper for interpretation and documentation in the patient's chart. The recorder-transmitter uses two types of electrodes applied to the finger and chest. These electrodes produce ECG tracings similar to those of a standard 12-lead ECG.

Credit card–size recorder

One recently developed recorder operates on a battery and is about the size of a credit card. When a patient becomes symptomatic, he holds the back of the card firmly to the center of his chest and pushes the start button. Four electrodes located on the back of the card sense electrical activity and record it. The card can store 30 seconds of activity and can later transmit the recording across phone lines for evaluation by a clinician.

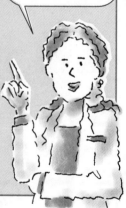

Now that's one heck of a charge card!

Havin' a heart wave

In a healthy heart, impulses originate in the sinoatrial node, travel through the atria to the atrioventricular node, and then to the ventricles. Most of the movement of the impulses is downward and to the left, the direction of a normal axis.

Swingin' on an axis

In an unhealthy heart, axis direction varies. That's because the direction of electrical activity swings away from areas of damage or

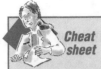

Axis direction in the heart

- With normal activity, impulses travel downward and to the left.
- The direction of electrical activity swings away from areas of damage or necrosis.
- The direction of electrical activity swings toward areas of hypertrophy.

A look at the leads

Each of the 12 leads views the heart from a different angle. These illustrations show the direction of each lead relative to the wave of depolarization (shown in color) and list the 12 views of the heart.

Views reflected on a 12-lead ECG	Leads	View of the heart
	Standard limb leads (bipolar)	
	I	lateral wall
	II	inferior wall
	III	inferior wall
	Augmented limb leads (unipolar)	
	aV_R	no specific view
	aV_L	lateral wall
	aV_F	inferior wall
	Precordial, or chest, leads (unipolar)	
	V_1	anteroseptal wall
	V_2	anteroseptal wall
	V_3	anterior and anteroseptal walls
	V_4	anterior wall
	V_5	lateral wall
	V_6	lateral wall

aV_R aV_L I   III   II aV_F

V_1 V_2 V_3 V_4 V_5 V_6

necrosis and toward areas of hypertrophy. Knowing the normal deflection of each lead will help you evaluate whether the electrical axis is normal or abnormal.

Obtaining a 12-lead ECG

You may be required to obtain an ECG in an emergency. To obtain the ECG, you'll need to:
• gather the appropriate supplies
• explain the procedure to the patient
• attach the electrodes properly
• know how to use an ECG machine
• interpret the recordings.
    Let's take a look at each aspect of the procedure.

Preparing for the recording

First, gather all the necessary supplies, including the ECG machine, recording paper, electrodes, and gauze pads. Take them to the patient's bedside. Then perform the following actions.

Explain the procedure

Next, tell the patient that the doctor has ordered an ECG, and explain the procedure. Emphasize that the test takes about 10 minutes and that it's a safe and painless way to evaluate cardiac function.

Answer the patient's questions, and offer reassurance. Preparing him well helps alleviate anxiety and promote cooperation.

Prepare the patient

Ask the patient to lie supine in the center of the bed with his arms at his sides. If he can't tolerate lying flat, raise the head of the bed to semi-Fowler's position. Ensure privacy, and expose the patient's arms, legs, and chest, draping him for comfort.

Select the electrode sites

Select the areas where you'll attach the electrodes. Choose spots that are flat and fleshy, not muscular or bony. Shave the area if it's excessively hairy. Clean excess oil or other substances from the skin to enhance electrode contact. Remember—the better the electrode contact, the better the recording.

Make the recording

The 12-lead ECG offers 12 different views of the heart, just as 12 photographers snapping the same picture would produce 12 different snapshots. To help ensure an accurate recording—or set of "pictures"—the electrodes must be applied correctly. Inaccurate placement of an electrode by greater than ⅗″ (1.5 cm) from its standardized position may lead to inaccurate waveforms and an incorrect ECG interpretation.

The 12-lead ECG requires four electrodes on the limbs and six across the front of the chest wall.

Going out on a limb lead

To record the bipolar limb leads I, II, and III and the unipolar limb leads aV_R, aV_L, and aV_F, place electrodes on both of the patient's arms and on his left leg. The right leg also receives an electrode, but that electrode acts as a ground and doesn't contribute to the waveform.

Where the wires go

Finding where to place the electrodes on the patient is easy because each leadwire is labeled or color coded. (See *Monitoring the limb leads*, pages 228 and 229.) For example, a wire—usually white—might be labeled "RA" for right arm. Another wire—usually red—might be labeled "LL" for left leg. Precordial leads are also labeled or color coded according to which wire corresponds to which lead.

No low leads allowed

To record the six precordial leads (V_1 through V_6), position the electrodes on specific areas of the anterior chest wall. (See *Positioning precordial electrodes*.) If they're placed too low, the ECG tracing will be inaccurate.

- Place lead V_1 over the fourth intercostal space at the right sternal border. To find the space, locate the sternal notch at the second rib and feel your way down along the sternal border until you reach the fourth intercostal space.
- Place lead V_2 just opposite V_1, over the fourth intercostal space at the left sternal border.
- Place lead V_3 midway between V_2 and V_4. *Tip:* Placing lead V_4 before lead V_3 makes it easier to see where to place lead V_3.
- Place lead V_4 over the fifth intercostal space at the left midclavicular line.
- Place lead V_5 over the fifth intercostal space at the left anterior axillary line.
- Place lead V_6 over the fifth intercostal space at the left midaxillary line. If you've placed leads V_4 through V_6 correctly, they should line up horizontally.

Give me more electrodes!

In addition to the 12-lead ECG, two other ECGs may be used for diagnostic purposes: the posterior-lead ECG and the right chest

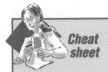

Cheat sheet

Placing the leads

- *Lead V_1:* Place over fourth intercostal space at the right sternal border.
- *Lead V_2:* Place over the fourth intercostal space at the left sternal border.
- *Lead V_3:* Place midway between leads V_2 and V_4.
- *Lead V_4:* Place over the fifth intercostal space at the left midclavicular line.
- *Lead V_5:* Place over the fifth intercostal space at the left anterior axillary line.
- *Lead V_6:* Place over the fifth intercostal space at the left midaxillary line.

Positioning precordial electrodes

The precordial leads complement the limb leads to provide a complete view of the heart. To record the precordial leads, place the electrodes as shown below.

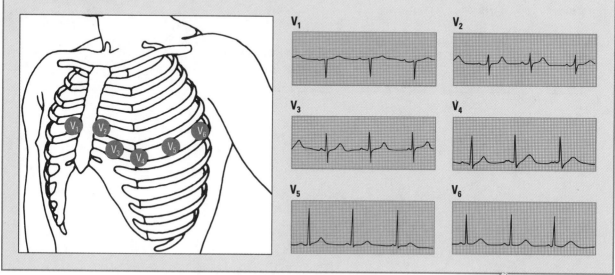

lead ECG. These ECGs use chest leads to assess areas standard 12-lead ECGs can't.

Seeing behind your back

Because of lung and muscle barriers, the usual chest leads can't "see" the heart's posterior surface to record myocardial damage there. Some doctors add three posterior leads to the 12-lead ECG: leads V_7, V_8, and V_9. These leads are placed opposite anterior leads V_4, V_5, and V_6, on the left side of the patient's back, following the same horizontal line.

On rare occasions, a doctor may request right-sided posterior leads. These leads are labeled V_7R, V_8R, and V_9R and are placed on the right side of the patient's back. Their placement is a mirror image of the electrodes on the left side of the back. This type of ECG provides information on the right posterior area of the heart.

Checking out the right chest

The usual 12-lead ECG evaluates only the left ventricle. If the right ventricle needs to be assessed for damage or dysfunction, the doctor may order a right chest lead ECG. For example, a patient with an inferior wall MI might have a right chest lead ECG to rule out

(Text continues on page 230.)

Cheat sheet

Seeing the heart's posterior surface

• Three posterior leads added to the 12-lead ECG: V_7, V_8, and V_9
• V_7, V_8, and V_9 opposite V_4, V_5, and V_6 on left side of back
• Right-sided posterior leads (V_7R, V_8R, V_9R) placed on right side of back (for information on right posterior of heart)

Monitoring the limb leads

These diagrams show electrode placement for the six limb leads. RA indicates right arm; LA, left arm; RL, right leg; and LL, left leg. The plus sign (+) indicates the positive pole, the minus sign (–) indicates the negative pole, and G indicates the ground. Below each diagram is a sample ECG recording for that lead.

Lead I
This lead connects the right arm (negative pole) with the left arm (positive pole).

Lead II
This lead connects the right arm (negative pole) with the left leg (positive pole).

Lead III
This lead connects the left arm (negative pole) with the left leg (positive pole).

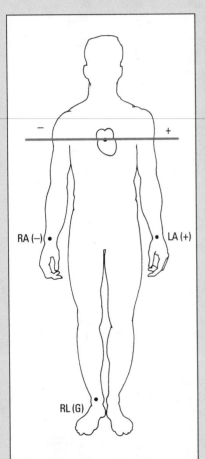

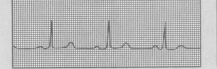

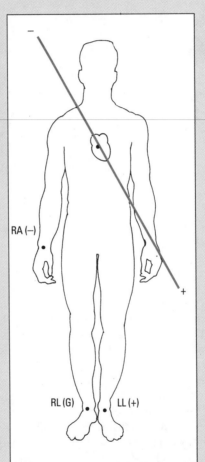

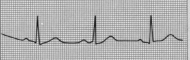

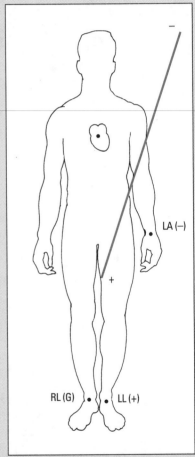

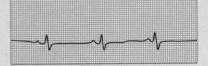

Lead aV_R
This lead connects the right arm (positive pole) with the heart (negative pole).

Lead aV_L
This lead connects the left arm (positive pole) with the heart (negative pole).

Lead aV_F
This lead connects the left leg (positive pole) with the heart (negative pole).

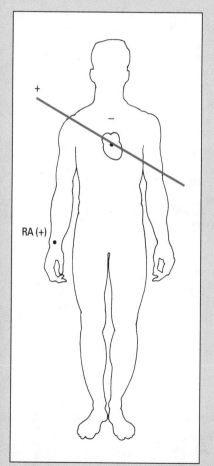

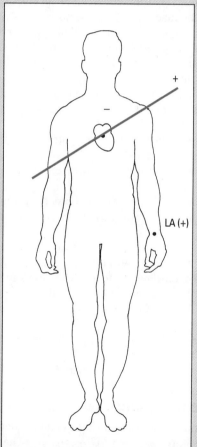

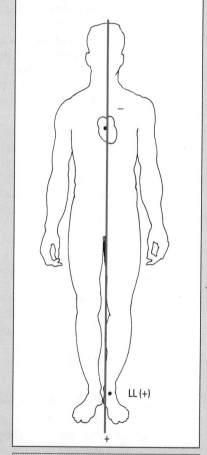

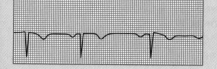

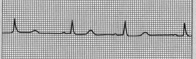

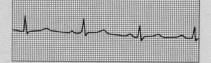

right ventricular involvement.

With this type of ECG, the six leads are placed on the right side of the chest in a mirror image of the standard precordial lead placement. Electrodes start at the left sternal border and swing down under the right breast area.

Know your machine

After you understand how to position the electrodes, familiarize yourself with the ECG machine. Machines come in two types: multichannel recorders and single-channel recorders.

With a multichannel recorder, you'll attach all electrodes to the patient at once and the machine prints a simultaneous view of all leads. With a single-channel recorder, you'll obtain a strip for one lead at a time by attaching and removing electrodes and stopping and starting the tracing each time. To begin recording the patient's ECG, follow these steps:

• Plug the cord of the ECG machine into a grounded outlet. If the machine operates on a charged battery, it may not need to be plugged in.

• Place one or all of the electrodes on the patient's chest, based on the type of machine you're using.

• Make sure all leads are securely attached, and then turn on the machine.

• Instruct the patient to relax, lie still, and breathe normally. Ask him not to talk during the recording to prevent distortion of the ECG tracing.

• Set the ECG paper speed selector to 25 mm/second. If necessary, enter the patient's identification data. Then calibrate or standardize the machine according to the manufacturer's instructions.

• Press the AUTO button and record the ECG. If you're performing a right chest lead ECG, select the appropriate button for recording.

• Observe the quality of the tracing. When the machine finishes the recording, turn it off.

• Remove the electrodes, and clean the patient's skin.

Interpreting the recording

ECG tracings from multichannel and single-channel machines look the same. (See *Multichannel ECG recording*.) The printout will show the patient's name and room number and, possibly, his medical record number. At the top of the printout, you'll see the patient's heart rate and wave durations, measured in seconds.

Some machines are also capable of recording ST-segment elevation and depression. The name of the lead will appear next to each 6-second strip.

Get out your pen

Be sure to write this information on the printout: date, time, doctor's name, and special circumstances. For example, you might record an episode of chest pain, abnormal electrolyte level, related drug treatment, abnormal placement of the electrodes, or the presence of an artificial pacemaker and whether a magnet was used while the ECG was obtained.

Remember, ECGs are legal documents. They belong on the patient's chart and must be saved for future reference and comparison with baseline strips.

Multichannel ECG recording

The top of a 12-lead ECG recording usually shows patient identification information along with the interpretation done by the machine. A rhythm strip is commonly included at the bottom of the recording.

Standardization

Look for the standardization marks on the recording, normally 10 small squares high. If the patient has high voltage complexes, the marks will be half as high. You'll also notice that lead markers separate the lead recordings on the paper and that each lead is labeled.

Also familiarize yourself with the order in which the leads are arranged on the ECG tracing. Getting accustomed to the layout of the tracing will help you interpret the ECG more quickly and accurately.

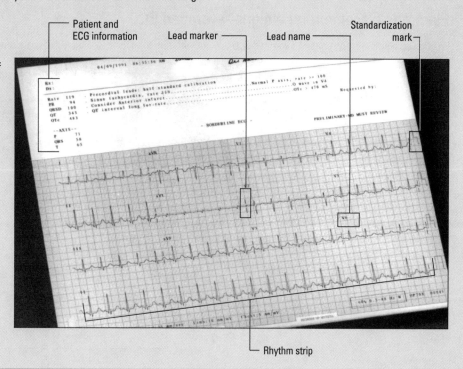

Patient and ECG information   Lead marker   Lead name   Standardization mark

Rhythm strip

Signal-averaged ECG

Although most patients will be tested with a 12-lead ECG, some may benefit from being tested with a signal-averaged ECG. This simple, noninvasive test helps identify patients at risk for sudden death from sustained ventricular tachycardia.

The test uses a computer to identify late electrical potentials—tiny impulses that follow normal depolarization. Late electrical potentials can't be detected by a 12-lead ECG.

Who gets the signal?

Patients prone to ventricular tachycardia—those who have had a recent MI or unexplained syncope, for example—are good candidates for a signal-averaged ECG. Keep in mind that a 12-lead ECG should be done when the patient is free from arrhythmias.

Noise free

A signal-averaged ECG is a noise-free, surface ECG recording taken from three specialized leads for several hundred heartbeats.

Electrode placement for a signal-averaged ECG

Positioning electrodes for a signal-averaged ECG is much different than for a 12-lead ECG. Here's one method.

1. Place the positive X electrode at the left fourth intercostal space, midaxillary line.
2. Place the negative X electrode at the right fourth intercostal space, midaxillary line.
3. Place the positive Y electrode at the left iliac crest.
4. Place the negative Y electrode at the superior aspect of the manubrium of the sternum.
5. Place the positive Z electrode at the fourth intercostal space left of the sternum.
6. Place the ground (G) on the lower right at the eighth rib.
7. Reposition the patient on his side, or have him sit forward. Then place the negative Z electrode on his back (not shown), directly posterior to the positive Z electrode.
8. Attach all the leads to the electrodes, being careful not to dislodge the posterior lead.
Now, you can obtain the tracing.

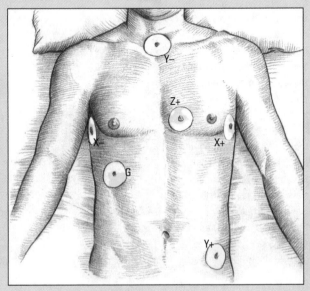

(See *Electrode placement for a signal-averaged ECG.*) The test takes approximately 10 minutes. The machine's computer detects late electrical potentials and then enlarges them so they're recognizable. The electrodes for a signal-averaged ECG are labeled X–, X+, Y–, Y+, Z–, Z+, and ground.

The machine averages signals from these leads to produce one representative QRS complex without artifacts. This process cancels noise, electrical impulses that don't occur as a repetitious pattern or with the same consistent timing as the QRS complex. That additional noise is filtered out so late electrical potentials can be detected. Muscle noise can't be filtered, however, so the patient must lie still for the test.

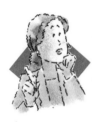

Quick quiz

1. The precordial leads are placed on the:
   A. anterior chest starting with the fourth intercostal space at the right sternal border.
   B. lateral chest starting with the fourth intercostal space at the left midaxillary line.
   C. posterior chest wall starting with the fourth intercostal space at the midscapular line.

Answer: A. Lead V_1 is placed anteriorly between the fourth and fifth ribs at the right sternal border. Leads V_2 to V_6 are then placed accordingly.

2. A signal-averaged ECG measures:
   A. electrical impulses from the SA node.
   B. late electrical potentials throughout the heart.
   C. action potentials of individual cardiac cells.

Answer: B. Signal-averaged ECGs measure late electrical potentials, tiny electrical impulses that occur after depolarization and can cause ventricular tachycardia.

3. A posterior-lead ECG is used to assess:
   A. posterior myocardial damage.
   B. inferior myocardial damage.
   C. damage to the interventricular septum.

Answer: A. This ECG assesses damage to the posterior surface of the heart, an area a standard 12-lead ECG can't detect.

4. The difference between a multichannel 12-lead ECG and a single-channel ECG is that a single-channel ECG:

    A.   requires 15 leads.

    B.   can't be used at the bedside.

    C.   requires rearranging electrodes for each lead.

Answer: C. A single-channel ECG must be obtained lead by lead.

5. A 12-lead ECG is used to assess function of the:

    A.   right ventricle.

    B.   left ventricle.

    C.   right and left ventricle simultaneously.

Answer: B. A 12-lead ECG gives a more complete view of the heart's electrical activity than a rhythm strip and is used to assess left ventricular function.

Scoring

☆☆☆   If you answered all five questions correctly, great job! You're the new leader of the 12-lead ECG pack!

☆☆   If you answered three or four correctly, we're impressed! Your leadership qualities are obvious, and you're next in line for a top job!

☆   If you answered fewer than three correctly, that's cool. You're a promising leader-in-training.

12

Interpreting a 12-lead ECG

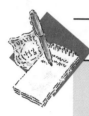

Just the facts

This chapter describes how to interpret a 12-lead ECG. By providing 12 different views of the heart's electrical activity, this test helps diagnose serious cardiac conditions. In this chapter, you'll learn:

♦ how to examine each lead's waveforms for abnormalities

♦ how to determine the heart's electrical axis

♦ what ECG changes occur in the patient with angina

♦ how to differentiate the types of acute myocardial infarction using a 12-lead ECG

♦ what 12-lead ECG changes occur with a bundle-branch block.

A look at interpreting a 12-lead ECG

To interpret a 12-lead ECG, use the systematic approach outlined here. Try to compare the patient's previous ECG with this one, if available. This will help you identify changes.

Check the ECG tracing to see if it's technically correct. Make sure the baseline is free from electrical interference and drift.

Scan the limb leads I, II, and III. The R-wave voltage in lead II should equal the sum of the R-wave voltage in leads I and III. Lead aV_R is typically negative. If these rules aren't met, the tracing may be recorded incorrectly.

Locate the lead markers on the waveform. Lead markers are the points where one lead changes to another.

Check the standardization markings to make sure all leads were recorded with the ECG machine's amplitude at the same setting. Standardization markings are usually located at the beginning of the strip.

Assess the heart rate and rhythm as you learned in earlier chapters.

Determine the heart's electrical axis. Use either the quadrant method or the degree method, described later in this chapter.

Examine limb leads I, II, and III. The R wave in lead II should be taller than in lead I. The waves in lead III should be smaller versions of the waves in lead I. The P wave or QRS complex may be inverted. Each lead should have flat ST segments and upright T waves, and pathologic Q waves should be absent.

Examine limb leads aV_L, aV_F, and aV_R. The tracings from leads aV_L and aV_F should be similar, but lead aV_F should have taller P and R waves. Lead aV_R has little diagnostic value. Its P wave, QRS complex, and T wave should be deflected downward.

Examine the R wave in the precordial leads. Normally, the R wave—the first positive deflection of the QRS complex—gets progressively taller from lead V_1 to lead V_5. Then it gets slightly smaller in lead V_6. (See *R-wave progression*.)

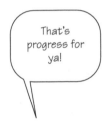

That's progress for ya!

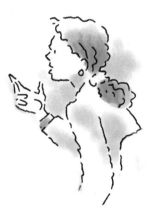

R-wave progression

These waveforms show normal R-wave progression through the precordial leads. Note that the R wave is the first positive deflection in the QRS complex. Also note that the S wave gets smaller, or regresses, from lead V_1 to V_6 until it finally disappears.

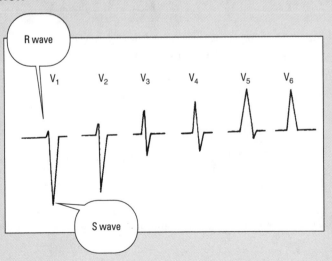

R wave

V_1 V_2 V_3 V_4 V_5 V_6

S wave

Examine the S wave—the negative deflection after an R wave—in the precordial leads. It appears extremely deep in lead V_1 and becomes progressively more shallow, usually disappearing at lead V_5.

All about waves

As you examine each lead, note where changes occur so you can identify the area of the heart affected. Remember that P waves should be upright; however, they may be inverted in lead aV_R or biphasic or inverted in leads III, aV_L, and V_1.

PR intervals should always be constant, just like QRS-complex durations. QRS-complex deflections will vary in different leads. Observe for pathologic Q waves.

Elevated one minute, depressed the next

ST segments should be isoelectric or have minimal deviation. ST-segment elevation greater than 1 mm above the baseline and ST-segment depression greater than 0.5 mm below the baseline are considered abnormal. Leads facing an injured area will have ST-segment elevations, and leads facing away will display ST-segment depressions.

That old, changeable T wave

The T wave normally deflects upward in leads I, II, and V_3 through V_6. It's inverted in lead aV_R and variable in the other leads. T-wave changes have many causes and aren't always a reason for alarm. Excessively tall, flat, or inverted T waves occurring with symptoms such as chest pain indicate ischemia.

Split-second duration

A normal Q wave generally has a duration of less than 0.04 second. An abnormal Q wave has either a duration of 0.04 second or more, a depth greater than 4 mm, or a height one-fourth of the R wave.

Abnormal Q waves indicate myocardial necrosis. These waves develop when depolarization can't take its normal path due to damaged tissue in the area. Remember that lead aV_R normally has a large Q wave, so disregard this lead when searching for abnormal Q waves.

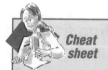

Cheat sheet

Looking at the waves

- *P waves:* upright; may be inverted in lead aV_R or biphasic or inverted in leads III, aV_L, and V_1
- *PR intervals:* always constant, like QRS-complex durations
- *QRS-complex deflections:* vary in different leads
- *Q waves:* may be pathologic; has a duration of less than 0.4 second when normal
- *T wave:* normally deflects upward in leads I, II, and V_3 through V_6; inverted in lead aV_R; variable in other leads
- *ST segments:* should be isoelectric or have minimal deviation

Finding the electrical axis

The electrical axis is the average direction of the heart's electrical activity during ventricular depolarization. Leads placed on the body sense the sum of the heart's electrical activity and record it as waveforms.

Cross my heart

You can determine your patient's electrical axis by examining the waveforms recorded from the six frontal plane leads: I, II, III, aV_R, aV_L, and aV_F. Imaginary lines drawn from each of the leads inter-

Hexaxial reference system

The hexaxial reference system consists of six bisecting lines, each representing one of the six limb leads, and a circle, representing the heart. The intersection of all lines divides the circle into equal, 30-degree segments.

Shifting degrees

Note that +0 degrees appears at the 3 o'clock position (positive pole lead I). Moving counterclockwise, the degrees become increasingly negative, until reaching ±180 degrees, at the 9 o'clock position (negative pole lead I).

    The bottom half of the circle contains the corresponding positive degrees. However, a positive-degree designation doesn't necessarily mean that the pole is positive.

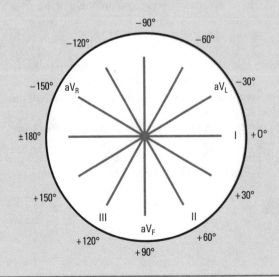

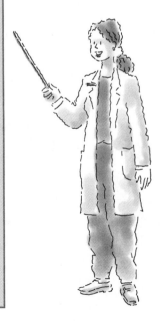

sect the center of the heart and form a diagram known as the hexaxial reference system. (See *Hexaxial reference system.*)

Where the axis falls

An axis that falls between 0 and +90 degrees is considered normal. An axis between +90 and +180 degrees indicates right axis deviation, and one between 0 and –90 degrees indicates left axis deviation. An axis between –180 and –90 degrees indicates extreme axis deviation and is called an indeterminate axis.

To determine your patient's electrical axis, use one of the two methods described here, the quadrant method or the degree method.

Quadrant method

The quadrant method, a fast, easy way to plot the heart's axis, involves observing the main deflection of the QRS complex in leads I and aV_F. (See *Quadrant method*, page 240.) Lead I indicates whether impulses are moving to the right or left, and lead aV_F indicates whether they're moving up or down.

If the QRS-complex deflection is positive or upright in both leads, the electrical axis is normal. If lead I is upright and lead aV_F points down, left axis deviation exists.

Right on and right in

When lead I points downward and lead aV_F is upright, right axis deviation exists. Both waves pointing down signal extreme axis deviation.

Degree method

A more precise axis calculation, the degree method gives an exact degree measurement of the electrical axis. (See *Degree method*, page 241.) It also allows you to determine the axis even if the QRS complex isn't clearly positive or negative in leads I and aV_F. To use this method, follow these steps.

Review all six leads, and identify the one that contains either the smallest QRS complex or the complex with an equal deflection above and below the baseline.

Use the hexaxial diagram to identify the lead perpendicular to this lead. For example, if lead I has the smallest QRS complex, then the lead perpendicular to the line representing lead I would be lead aV_F.

After you've identified the perpendicular lead, examine its QRS complex. If the electrical activity is moving toward the posi-

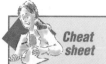

Determining the electrical axis

- Examine the waveforms from the six frontal place leads: I, II, III, aV_R, aV_L, and aV_F.
- Axis between 0 and +90 degrees is normal.
- Axis between +90 and +180 degrees indicates a right axis deviation.
- Axis between 0 and –90 degrees indicates a left axis deviation.
- Axis between –180 and –90 degrees indicates an extreme axis deviation.

Quadrant method

This chart will help you quickly determine the direction of a patient's electrical axis. Just observe the deflections of the QRS complexes in leads I and aV$_F$. Then check the chart to determine whether the patient's axis is normal or has a left, right, or extreme axis deviation.

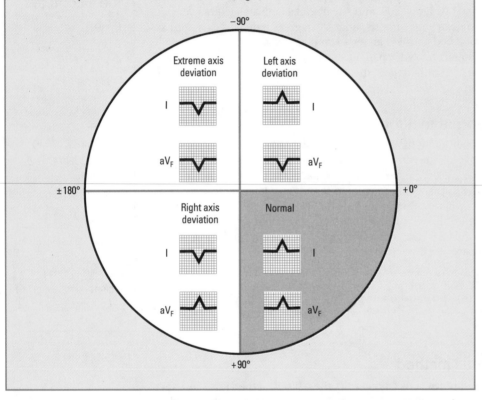

Memory jogger

Think of the QRS-complex deflections in leads I and aV$_F$ as thumbs pointing up or down. Two thumbs up is normal; anything else is abnormal.

tive pole of a lead, the QRS complex deflects upward. If it's moving away from the positive pole of a lead, the QRS complex deflects downward.

Plot this information on the hexaxial diagram to determine the direction of the electrical axis.

Axis deviation

Finding a patient's electrical axis can help confirm a diagnosis or narrow the range of possible diagnoses. (See *Causes of axis deviation*, page 242.) Factors that influence the location of the axis include the heart's position in the chest, the heart's size, the patient's

Degree method

The degree method of determining axis deviation allows you to identify a patient's electrical axis by degrees on the hexaxial system, not just by quadrant. To use this method, take the following steps.

Step 1
Identify the lead with the smallest QRS complex or the equiphasic QRS complex. In this example, it's lead III.

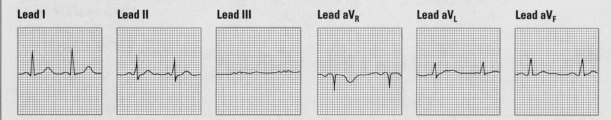

| Lead I | Lead II | Lead III | Lead aV$_R$ | Lead aV$_L$ | Lead aV$_F$ |

Step 2
Locate the axis for lead III on the hexaxial diagram. Then find the axis perpendicular to it, which is the axis for lead aV$_R$.

Step 3
Now, examine the QRS complex in lead aV$_R$, noting whether the deflection is positive or negative. As you can see, the QRS complex for this lead is negative. This tells you that the electric current is moving toward the negative pole of aV$_R$, which, on the hexaxial diagram, is in the right lower quadrant at +30 degrees. So the electrical axis here is normal at +30 degrees.

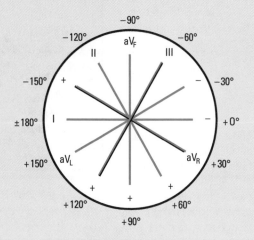

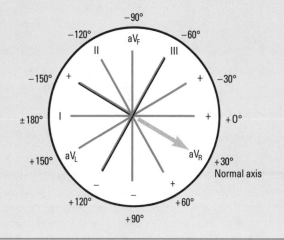

body size or type, the conduction pathways, and the force of the electrical impulses being generated.

Remember that electrical activity in the heart swings away from areas of damage or necrosis, so the damaged part of the heart will be the last area to be depolarized. For example, in right bundle-branch block, the impulse travels quickly down the normal left side and then moves slowly down the right side. This shifts the electrical forces to the right, causing right axis deviation.

No worries

Axis deviation isn't always cause for alarm, and it isn't always cardiac in origin. For example, infants and children normally have right axis deviation. Pregnant women normally have left axis deviation.

Disorders affecting 12-lead ECGs

A 12-lead ECG is used to diagnose such conditions as angina, bundle-branch block, and myocardial infarction (MI). By reviewing sample ECGs, you'll know what classic signs to look for. Here's a rundown on those three common cardiac conditions and what 12-lead ECG signs to look for.

Angina

During an episode of angina, the myocardium demands more oxygen than the coronary arteries can deliver. The arteries are unable to deliver enough blood, most often as a result of a narrowing of the arteries from coronary artery disease (CAD), a condition that may be complicated by platelet clumping, thrombus formation, or vasospasm.

An episode of angina usually lasts between 2 and 10 minutes. The closer to 30 minutes the pain lasts, the more likely the pain is from an MI rather than angina.

Stable or unstable?

You may hear the term stable angina applied to certain conditions and unstable angina applied to others. In stable angina, pain is triggered by exertion or stress and is often relieved by rest. Each episode follows the same pattern.

Unstable angina, on the other hand, is more easily provoked, often waking the patient. It's also unpredictable and worsens over time. The patient with unstable angina is treated as a medical emergency. The onset of unstable angina often portends an MI.

In addition to the ECG changes noted below, the patient with unstable angina will complain of chest pain that may radiate. The pain is generally more intense and lasts longer than the pain of

Causes of axis deviation

This list covers common causes of right and left axis deviation.

Left
• Normal variation
• Inferior wall myocardial infarction (MI)
• Left anterior hemiblock
• Wolff-Parkinson-White syndrome
• Mechanical shifts (ascites, pregnancy, tumors)
• Left bundle-branch block
• Left ventricular hypertrophy
• Aging

Right
• Normal variation
• Lateral wall MI
• Left posterior hemiblock
• Right bundle-branch block
• Emphysema
• Right ventricular hypertrophy

stable angina. The patient may also be pale, clammy, nauseous, and anxious.

Fleeting change of heart

Most patients with either form of angina show ischemic changes on the ECG only during the angina attack. (See *ECG changes associated with angina.*) Because these changes may be fleeting, always obtain an order for, and perform, a 12-lead ECG as soon as the patient reports chest pain.

The ECG will allow you to analyze all parts of the heart and pinpoint which area and coronary artery are involved. By recognizing danger early, you may be able to prevent an MI or even death.

Drugs are a key component of anginal treatment and may include nitrates, beta-adrenergic blockers, calcium channel blockers, and aspirin or glycoprotein IIb/IIIa inhibitors to reduce platelet aggregation.

Bundle-branch block

One potential complication of an MI is a bundle-branch block. In this disorder, either the left or the right bundle branch fails to conduct impulses. A bundle-branch block that occurs farther down the left bundle, in the posterior or anterior fasciculus, is called a hemiblock.

ECG changes associated with angina

Here are some classic ECG changes involving the T wave and ST segment that you may see when monitoring a patient with angina.

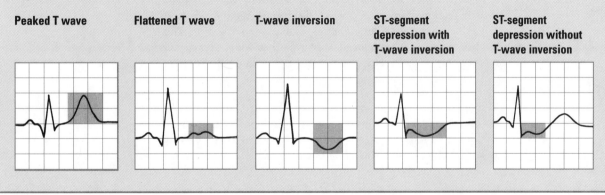

| Peaked T wave | Flattened T wave | T-wave inversion | ST-segment depression with T-wave inversion | ST-segment depression without T-wave inversion |

Some blocks require treatment with a temporary pacemaker. Others are monitored only to detect whether they progress to a more complete block.

Impulsive behavior

In a bundle-branch block, the impulse travels down the unaffected bundle branch and then from one myocardial cell to the next to depolarize the ventricle.

Because this cell-to-cell conduction progresses much more slowly than the conduction along the specialized cells of the conduction system, ventricular depolarization is prolonged.

Wide world of complexes

Prolonged ventricular depolarization means that the QRS complex will be widened. The normal width of the complex is 0.06 to 0.10 second. If the width increases to greater than 0.12 second, a bundle-branch block is present.

After you identify a bundle-branch block, examine lead V_1, which lies to the right of the heart, and lead V_6, which lies to the left of the heart. You'll use these leads to determine whether the block is in the right or the left bundle.

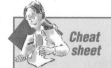

Cheat sheet

Determining bundle-branch block

- *QRS complex:* width increases to greater than 0.12 second with bundle-branch block
- *Lead V_1 (to right of heart) and V_6 (to left of heart):* used to determine whether block is in right or left bundle

Right bundle-branch block

Right bundle-branch block (RBBB) occurs with conditions, such as anterior wall MI, CAD, and pulmonary embolism. It may also occur without cardiac disease. If this block develops as the heart rate increases, it's called rate-related RBBB. (See *How RBBB occurs.*)

In this disorder, the QRS complex is greater than 0.12 second and has a different configuration, sometimes resembling rabbit ears or the letter "M." (See *Recognizing RBBB*, page 246.) Septal depolarization isn't affected in lead V_1, so the initial small R wave remains.

The R wave is followed by an S wave, which represents left ventricular depolarization, and a tall R wave (called R prime, or R'), which represents late right ventricular depolarization. The T wave is negative in this lead. However, that deflection is called a secondary T-wave change and is of no clinical significance.

Opposing moves

The opposite occurs in lead V_6. A small Q wave is followed by depolarization of the left ventricle, which produces a tall R wave. Depolarization of the right ventricle then causes a broad S wave. In lead V_6, the T wave should be positive.

How RBBB occurs

In right bundle-branch block (RBBB), the initial impulse activates the interventricular septum from left to right, just as in normal activation (arrow 1). Next, the left bundle branch activates the left ventricle (arrow 2). The impulse then crosses the interventricular septum to activate the right ventricle (arrow 3).

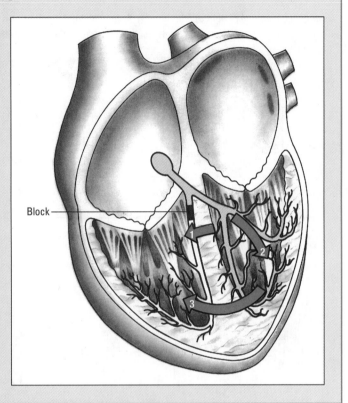

Block

Left bundle-branch block

Left bundle-branch block (LBBB) never occurs normally. This block is usually caused by hypertensive heart disease, aortic stenosis, degenerative changes of the conduction system, or CAD. (See *How LBBB occurs*, page 247.) When it occurs along with an anterior wall MI, it usually signals complete heart block, which requires insertion of a pacemaker.

One ventricle after another

In LBBB, the QRS complex will be greater than 0.12 second because the ventricles are activated sequentially, not simultaneously. (See *Recognizing LBBB*, page 248.) As the wave of depolarization spreads from the right ventricle to the left, a wide S wave is produced in lead V_1, with a positive T wave. The S wave may be preceded by a Q wave or a small R wave.

Recognizing RBBB

This 12-lead ECG shows the characteristic changes of right bundle-branch block (RBBB). In lead V_1, note the rsR′ pattern and T-wave inversion. In lead V_6, see the widened S wave and the upright T wave. Also note the prolonged QRS complexes.

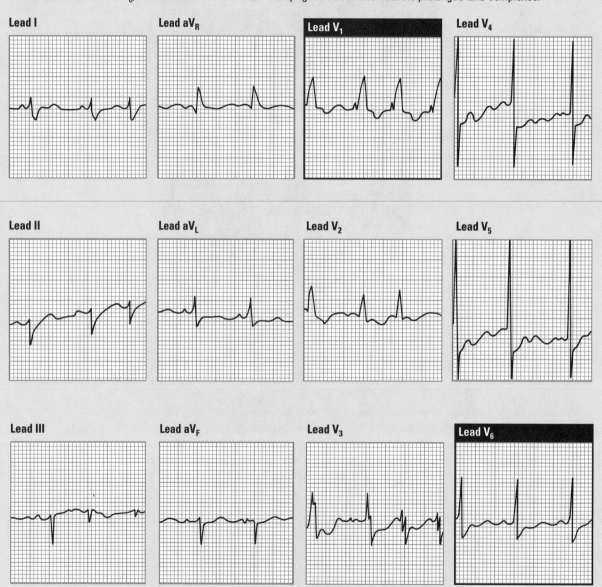

How LBBB occurs

In left bundle-branch block (LBBB), the impulse first travels down the right bundle branch (arrow 1). Then the impulse activates the interventricular septum from right to left (arrow 2), the opposite of normal activation. Finally, the impulse activates the left ventricle (arrow 3).

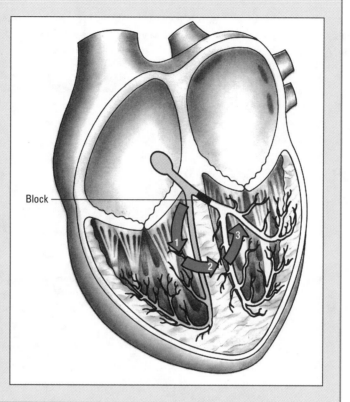

Block

Slurring your R waves

In lead V_6, no initial Q wave occurs. A tall, notched R wave, or a slurred one, is produced as the impulse spreads from right to left. This initial positive deflection is a sign of LBBB. The T wave is negative.

Myocardial infarction

Unlike angina, pain from an MI lasts for at least 20 minutes, may persist for several hours, and is unrelieved by rest. MI usually occurs in the left ventricle, although the location may vary depending on the coronary artery affected.

For as long as the myocardium is deprived of an oxygen-rich blood supply, an ECG will reflect the three pathologic changes of an MI: ischemia, injury, and infarction. (See *Reciprocal changes in an MI*, page 249.)

(Text continues on page 250.)

Recognizing LBBB

This 12-lead ECG shows characteristic changes of left bundle-branch block (LBBB). All leads have prolonged QRS complexes. In lead V_1, note the QS wave pattern. In lead V_6, you'll see the slurred R wave and T-wave inversion. The elevated ST segments and upright T waves in leads V_1 to V_4 are also common in LBBB.

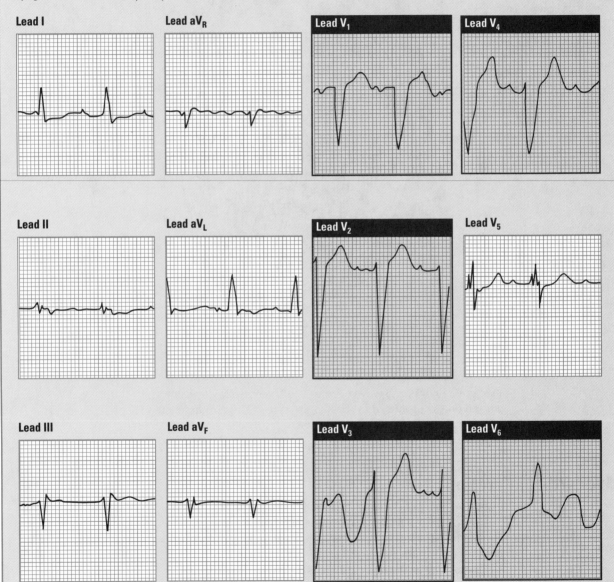

Reciprocal changes in an MI

Ischemia, injury, and infarction—the three I's of a myocardial infarction (MI)—produce characteristic ECG changes. Changes shown by the leads that reflect electrical activity in damaged areas are shown on the right.

Reciprocal leads, those opposite the damaged area, will show opposite ECG changes, as shown to the left of the illustration.

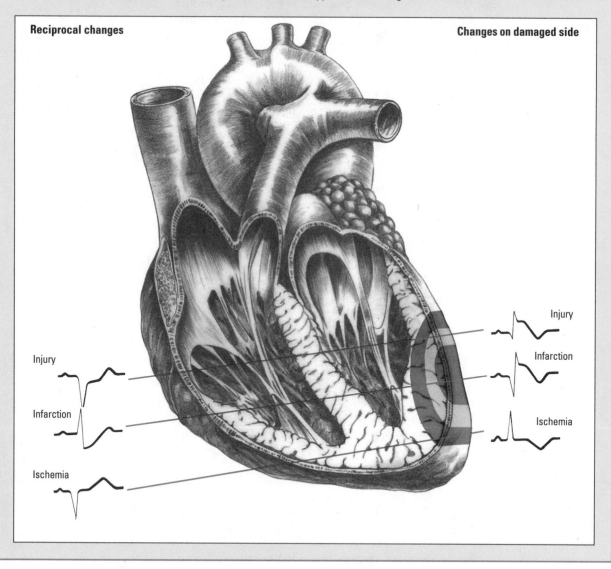

Reciprocal changes

Changes on damaged side

Injury

Infarction

Ischemia

Injury

Infarction

Ischemia

Zone of infarction

The area of myocardial necrosis is called the zone of infarction. Scar tissue eventually replaces the dead tissue, and the damage caused is irreversible.

The ECG change associated with a necrotic area is a pathologic Q wave, which results from lack of depolarization. Such Q waves are permanent. MIs that don't produce Q waves are called non–Q-wave MIs.

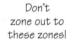

Don't zone out to these zones!

Zone of injury

The zone of infarction is surrounded by the zone of injury, which shows up on an ECG as an elevated ST segment. ST-segment elevation results from a prolonged lack of blood supply.

Zone of ischemia

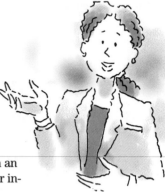

The outermost area is called the zone of ischemia and results from an interrupted blood supply. This zone is represented on an ECG by T-wave inversion. Changes in the zones of ischemia or injury are reversible.

From ischemia to injury

Generally, as an MI occurs, the patient experiences chest pain and an ECG shows changes, such as ST-segment elevation, which indicates that myocardial injury is occurring. You'll also typically see T waves flatten and become inverted.

Rapid treatment can prevent myocardial necrosis. However, if symptoms persist for more than 6 hours, little can be done to prevent necrosis. That's one of the reasons patients are advised to seek medical attention as soon as symptoms begin.

The telltale Q wave

Q waves can appear hours to days after an MI and signify that an entire thickness of the myocardium has become necrotic. Tall R waves in reciprocal leads can also develop. This type of MI is called a transmural, or Q-wave, MI.

Back to baseline

Knowing how long such changes last can help you determine how long ago an MI occurred. ST segments return to baseline within a few days to 2 weeks. Inverted T waves may persist for several months. Although not every patient who has had an MI develops Q waves, those who do have them on their ECGs indefinitely.

What to do for an MI

The most important thing you can do for a patient with an MI is to remain vigilant about detecting changes in his condition and in his ECG. (See *Monitoring MI patients.*)

The primary goal of treatment for an MI is to limit the size of the infarction by decreasing cardiac workload and increasing oxygen supply to the myocardium. (See *Improving blood flow.*) In addition to rest, pain relief, and supplemental oxygen, such medications as nitroglycerin, morphine sulfate, beta-adrenergic blockers, calcium channel blockers, angiotensin-converting enzyme inhibitors, and antiarrhythmics are used. Aspirin or glycoprotein IIb/IIIa inhibitors may be used to reduce platelet aggregation. Thrombolytic therapy also may be prescribed to dissolve a thrombus occluding a coronary artery.

Identifying types of MI

The location of the MI is a critical factor in determining the most appropriate treatment and predicting probable complications. Characteristic ECG changes that occur with each type of MI are localized to the leads overlying the infarction site. (See *Locating myocardial damage*, page 252.) Here's a look at characteristic ECG changes that occur with different types of MIs.

Anterior wall MI

The left anterior descending artery supplies blood to the anterior portion of the left ventricle. The artery supplies blood to the ven-

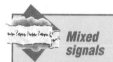

Mixed signals

Monitoring MI patients

Remember that specific leads monitor specific walls of the heart. Here's a quick overview of those leads.

- For an anterior wall MI, monitor lead V_1 or MCL_1.
- For a septal wall MI, monitor lead V_1 or MCL_1 to pick up hallmark changes.
- For a lateral wall MI, monitor lead V_6 or MCL_6.
- For an inferior wall MI, monitor lead II.

Improving blood flow

Increasing the blood supply to the heart of a patient who has had an MI can help prevent further damage to his heart. In addition to medications, blood flow to the heart can be improved by:
- intra-aortic balloon pump
- percutaneous transluminal coronary angioplasty
- atherectomy
- laser treatment
- stent placement
- coronary artery bypass graft.

Locating myocardial damage

After you've noted characteristic lead changes of an acute myocardial infarction, use this chart to identify the areas of damage. Match the lead changes in the second column with the affected wall in the first column and the artery involved in the third column. Column four shows reciprocal lead changes.

Wall affected	Leads	Artery involved	Reciprocal changes
Inferior (diaphragmatic)	II, III, aV$_F$	Right coronary artery	I, aV$_L$ and, possibly, V$_4$
Lateral	I, aV$_L$, V$_5$, V$_6$	Circumflex artery, branch of left coronary artery	V$_1$, V$_2$
Anterior	V$_2$ to V$_4$	Left coronary artery, LAD artery	II, III, aV$_F$
Posterior	V$_1$, V$_2$	Right coronary artery, circumflex artery	R wave greater than S wave in V$_1$ and V$_2$; depressed ST segments; elevated T wave
Anterolateral	I, aV$_L$, V$_4$ to V$_6$	LAD artery, circumflex artery	II, III, aV$_F$
Anteroseptal	V$_1$ to V$_3$	LAD artery	None
Right ventricular	V$_4$R, V$_5$R, V$_6$R	Right coronary artery	None

tricular septum and portions of the right and left bundle-branch systems.

When the anterior descending artery becomes occluded, an anterior wall MI occurs. (See *Recognizing an anterior wall MI.*) Complications of an anterior wall MI include varying second-degree atrioventricular blocks, bundle-branch blocks, ventricular irritability, and left-sided failure.

Changing the leads

An anterior wall MI causes characteristic ECG changes in leads V$_2$ to V$_4$. The precordial leads show poor R-wave progression because the left ventricle can't depolarize normally. ST-segment elevation and T-wave inversion are also present.

The reciprocal leads for the anterior wall are the inferior leads II, III, and aV$_F$. They show tall R waves and depressed ST segments.

Recognizing an anterior wall MI

This 12-lead ECG shows typical characteristics of an anterior wall myocardial infarction (MI). Note that the R waves don't progress through the precordial leads. Also note the ST-segment elevation in leads V_2 and V_3. As expected, the reciprocal leads II, III, and aV_F show slight ST-segment depression. Axis deviation is normal at +60 degrees.

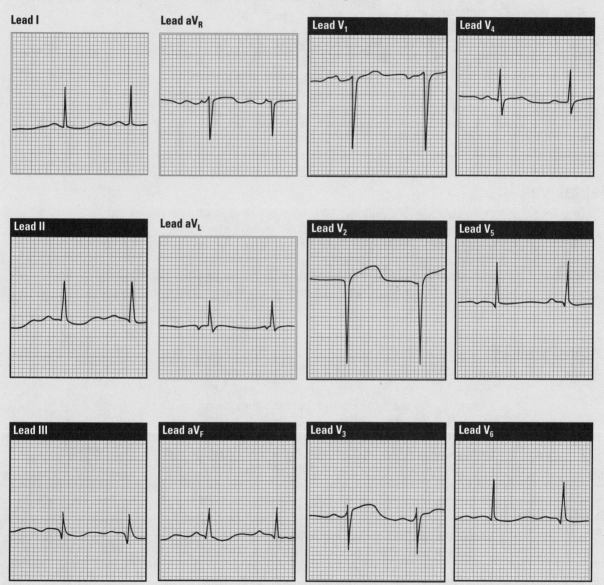

Cheat sheet

ECGs and different types of MIs

- *Anterior wall MI:* ECG changes in leads V_2 and V_4
- *Septal wall MI:* ECG changes in leads V_1 and V_2
- *Lateral wall MI:* changes in left lateral leads I, aV_L, and V_5 and V_6
- *Inferior wall MI:* ECG changes in the inferior leads II, III, and aV_F
- *Right ventricular MI:* ST-segment elevation, pathologic Q waves, and inverted T waves in right precordial leads V_2R to V_6R
- *Posterior wall MI:* tall R waves, ST-segment depression, upright T waves; obtain information about posterior wall and pathologic Q waves from leads V_7 to V_9 using a posterior ECG

Septal wall MI

The patient with a septal wall MI has an increased risk for developing a ventricular septal defect. ECG changes are present in leads V_1 and V_2. In those leads, the R wave disappears, the ST segment rises, and the T wave inverts.

Because the left anterior descending artery also supplies blood to the ventricular septum, a septal wall MI often accompanies an anterior wall MI.

Lateral wall MI

A lateral wall MI is usually caused by a blockage in the left circumflex artery and shows characteristic changes in the left lateral leads I, aV_L, V_5, and V_6. The reciprocal leads for a lateral wall infarction are V_1 and V_2.

This type of infarction typically causes premature ventricular contractions and varying degrees of heart block. A lateral wall MI usually accompanies an anterior or inferior wall MI.

Inferior wall MI

An inferior wall MI is usually caused by occlusion of the right coronary artery and produces characteristic ECG changes in the inferior leads II, III, and aV_F and reciprocal changes in the lateral leads I and aV_L. (See *Recognizing an inferior wall MI.*) It's also called a diaphragmatic MI because the inferior wall of the heart lies over the diaphragm.

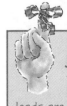

Memory jogger

To remember which leads are critical in diagnosing a lateral wall MI, think of the l's in lateral MI and left lateral leads.

Recognizing an inferior wall MI

This 12-lead ECG shows the characteristic changes of an inferior wall myocardial infarction (MI). In leads II, III, and aV$_F$, note the T-wave inversion, ST-segment elevation, and pathologic Q waves. In leads I and aV$_L$, note the slight ST-segment depression, a reciprocal change. This ECG shows left axis deviation at −60 degrees.

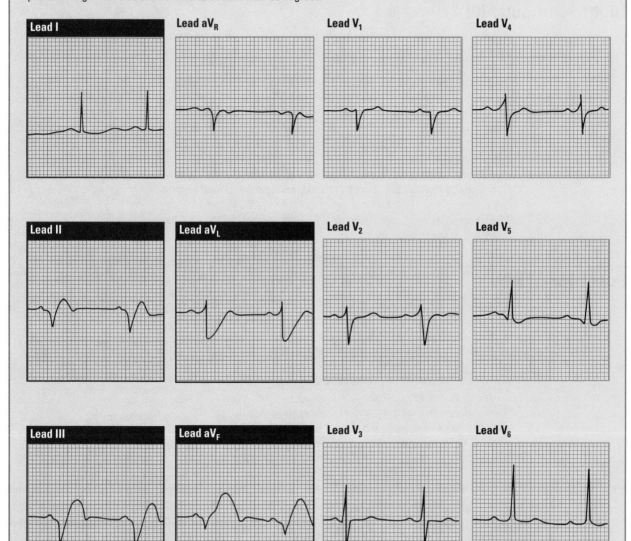

Patients with inferior wall MI are at risk for developing sinus bradycardia, sinus arrest, heart block, and premature ventricular contractions. This type of MI occurs alone, with a lateral wall MI, or with a right ventricular MI.

Right ventricular MI

A right ventricular MI usually follows occlusion of the right coronary artery. This type of MI rarely occurs alone. In fact, 40% of all patients with an inferior wall MI also suffer a right ventricular MI.

A right ventricular MI can lead to right ventricular failure or right-sided block. The classic changes are ST-segment elevation, pathologic Q waves, and inverted T waves in the right precordial leads V_2R to V_6R.

Take the right lead

Identifying a right ventricular MI is difficult without information from the right precordial leads. If these leads aren't available, you can observe leads II, III, and aV_F or watch leads V_1, V_2, and V_3 for ST elevation. If a right ventricular MI has occurred, use lead II to monitor for further damage.

Posterior wall MI

A posterior wall MI is caused by occlusion of either the right coronary artery or the left circumflex arteries. This MI produces reciprocal changes on leads V_1 and V_2.

Classic ECG changes in a posterior wall MI include tall
R waves, ST-segment depression, and upright T waves. Posterior infarctions usually accompany inferior infarctions. Information about the posterior wall and pathologic Q waves that might occur can be obtained from leads V_7 to V_9 using a posterior ECG.

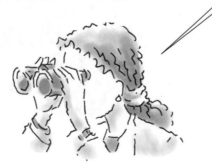

Identifying a right ventricular MI is difficult without information from the right precordial leads.

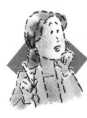

Quick quiz

1. Your patient's ECG shows positively deflected QRS complexes in leads I and aV_F. Using the four-quadrant method for determining the electrical axis, you determine that he has a:
A.   normal axis.
B.   left axis deviation.
C.   right axis deviation.

Answer: A. If the QRS-complex deflection is positive or upright in both leads, the electrical axis is normal.

2. Your patient's ECG shows a negatively deflected QRS complex in lead I and a positively deflected one in lead aV_F. Using the four-quadrant method for determining electrical axis, you determine that he has a:
A.   normal axis.
B.   left axis deviation.
C.   right axis deviation.

Answer: C. When lead I points downward and lead aV_F is upright, right axis deviation exists. Both waves pointing down signals indeterminate axis deviation.

3. If your patient has a T-wave inversion, ST-segment elevation, and pathologic Q waves in leads II, III, and aV_F, suspect an acute MI in the:
A.   anterior wall.
B.   inferior wall.
C.   lateral wall.

Answer: B. Leads II, III, and aV_F face the inferior wall of the left ventricle, so the ECG changes there are indicative of an acute inferior wall MI.

4. If a patient's QRS complex has an R′ wave in V_1, suspect:
A.   right ventricular hypertrophy.
B.   left ventricular hypertrophy.
C.   RBBB.

Answer: C. In RBBB, depolarization of the right ventricle takes longer than normal, thereby creating an R′ wave in lead V_1.

5. Myocardial injury is represented on an ECG by the presence of a:
A.   T-wave inversion.
B.   ST-segment elevation.
C.   pathologic Q wave.

Answer: B. ST-segment elevation is the ECG change that corresponds with myocardial injury. It's caused by a prolonged lack of blood supply.

6.   On a 12-lead ECG, a posterior wall infarction produces:
    A   deep, broad Q waves in leads V_1 through V_3.
    B.   inverse or mirror image changes in V_1 and V_2.
    C.   raised ST segments in all leads.

Answer: B. Leads V_1 and V_2 show reciprocal changes when a posterior wall MI occurs. Look at the mirror images of these leads to determine the presence of a posterior wall MI.

7.   The appearance of Q waves in the aftermath of an MI signify that:
    A.   the interventricular septum has become injured.
    B.   an entire thickness of the myocardium has become necrotic.
    C.   a superficial layer of the myocardium has become ischemic.

Answer: B. Q waves can appear hours to days after an MI and signify that an entire thickness of the myocardium has become necrotic.

8.   An ST segment located 1.5 mm above the baseline is considered:
    A.   normal.
    B.   slightly depressed.
    C.   abnormally elevated.

Answer: C. ST segments should be isoelectric or have minimal deviation. ST-segment elevation greater than 1 mm above the baseline is considered abnormal.

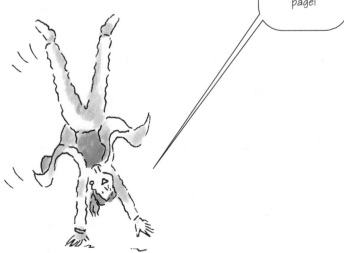

So far, so good. Now check out the strips on the next page!

Test strips

OK, it's time to try out a couple of test ECGs.

9. In the 12-lead ECG below, you'll see an rsR′ pattern in lead V_1, as well as T-wave inversion. Looking at lead V_6, you'll note a widened S wave and an upright T wave. These changes indicate:

    A.   right ventricular MI.

    B.   LBBB.

    C.   RBBB.

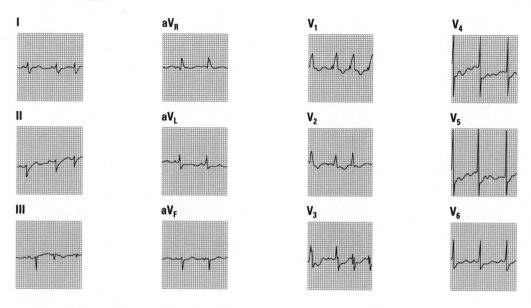

Answer: C. The rsR′ configuration in lead V_1 and the wide S wave in V_6 indicate RBBB.

10. Your patient says he thinks he might have had a heart attack about 3 years ago but, because he never went to the doctor, he doesn't know for sure. Looking at his admission ECG, you think he definitely had an MI at some point. You base your assessment on the presence of:

    A.   pathologic Q waves in leads II, III, and aV_F.

    B.   inverted T waves in leads I, aV_L, and V_6.

    C.   depressed ST segments in leads II, aV_L, and V_5.

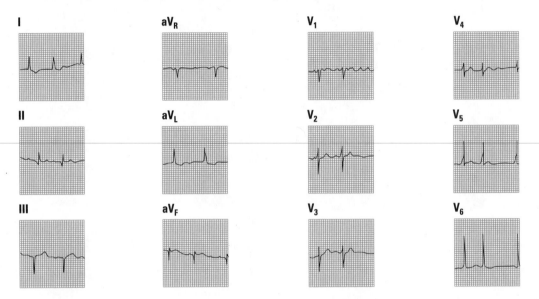

Answer: A. Old damage to the myocardium is indicated by the presence of pathologic Q waves, in this case in leads II, III, and aV_F. Those findings lead you to suspect the patient suffered an inferior wall MI at some point.

Scoring

☆☆☆ If you answered all ten questions correctly, wow! You've graduated (with honors) from the School of 12-Lead ECG Interpretation!

☆☆ If you answered six to nine correctly, super! You're ready to take a graduate course on 12-lead ECG interpretation!

☆ If you answered fewer than six correctly, you're definitely on the right track. Just review your notes from 12-Lead ECG Interpretation 101!

Appendices and index

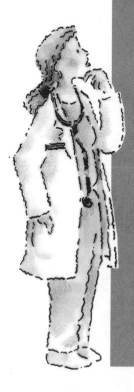

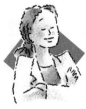

Practice makes perfect

1. You're caring for a patient with a history of mitral valve prolapse. Based on your knowledge of the heart's anatomy, you know that the mitral valve is located:
  A.   between the left atrium and the left ventricle.
  B.   where the left ventricle meets the aorta.
  C.   between the right atrium and right ventricle.

2. A 45-year-old patient is admitted to your floor for observation after undergoing cardiac catheterization. His test results reveal a blockage in the circumflex artery. The circumflex artery supplies oxygenated blood to which area of the heart?
  A.   Anterior wall of the left ventricle
  B.   Left atrium
  C.   Right bundle branch

3. Which of the following choices is responsible for slowing heart rate?
  A.   norepinephrine
  B.   Vagus nerve
  C.   epinephrine

4. Which cycle describes cardiac cells at rest?
  A.   Repolarization
  B.   Polarization
  C.   Depolarization

5. A patient admitted with an acute MI complains of chest pain. When you look at his ECG monitor you note a heart rate of 35 beats/minute. Which area of his heart has taken over as the heart's pacemaker?
  A.   SA node
  B.   AV node
  C.   Purkinje fibers

6. A 37-year-old patient comes to the emergency department complaining of chest pain that began while he was mowing the lawn. You immediately begin cardiac monitoring and administer oxygen. Next you obtain a 12-lead ECG. You know that the six limb leads you apply will give you information about what area of the patient's heart?
  A.   The frontal plane
  B.   The horizontal plane
  C.   The vertical plane

7. Which lead on a cardiac monitor is equivalent to V_1 on a 12-lead ECG?

    A.   Lead I

    B. MCL_6

    C. MCL_1

8. A patient with heart failure is transferred to your unit from the medical surgical floor. Before initiating cardiac monitoring you must first:

    A.   prepare the skin by rubbing it until it reddens.

    B.   press the adhesive edge around the outside of the electrode to the patient's chest.

    C.   press one side of the electrode against the patient's skin.

9. A 58-year-old patient is admitted with an acute MI that he suffered while shoveling snow. After you begin cardiac monitoring, you note a baseline that's thick and unreadable. How do you interpret this finding?

    A.   Electrical interference

    B.   Artifact

    C.   Wandering baseline

10. What does the horizontal axis of an ECG represent?

    A.   Amplitude

    B.   Time

    C.   Electrical voltage

11. A 65-year-old patient diagnosed with angina is admitted to your telemetry unit. You begin cardiac monitoring and record a rhythm strip. Using the 8-step method of rhythm strip interpretation, which of the following would you do first?

    A.   Calculate the heart rate.

    B.   Evaluate the P wave.

    C.   Check the rhythm.

12. A 72-year-old patient calls you to his room because he's experiencing substernal chest pain that radiates to his jaw. You record a rhythm strip and monitor his vital signs. Which portion of the patient's ECG complex may become elevated or depressed indicating myocardial damage?

    A.   T wave

    B.   ST segment

    C.   QRS complex

13. A 76-year-old patient with heart failure is receiving furosemide (Lasix) 40 mg I.V twice daily. When you look at her rhythm strip, you note prominent U waves. Which of the following conditions may have caused U waves to appear on your patient's rhythm strip?

    A.   Hypokalemia

    B.   Hypocalcemia

    C.   Worsening heart failure

14. An 80-year-old patient with a history of atrial fibrillation is admitted with digoxin toxicity. When you assess his rhythm strip using the 10-times method, you note that his heart rate is 40 beats/minute. Based on this finding you should:

    A.   check the patient's pulse and correlate it with the heart rate on the rhythm strip.

    B.   recheck the heart rate on the rhythm strip using the sequence method.

    C.   record another rhythm strip and reassess the heart rate on the rhythm strip.

15. A patient with a history of paroxysmal atrial tachycardia develops digoxin toxicity. Because digoxin toxicity may cause prolongation of the PR interval, you must monitor his rhythm strip closely. What's the duration of a normal PR interval?

    A.   0.06 to 0.10 second

    B.   0.12 to 0.20 second

    C.   0.36 to 0.44 second

16. A patient who has been taking digoxin (Lanoxin) suddenly develops the rhythm shown below. What's your interpretation of the rhythm?

    A.   Normal sinus rhythm

    B.   Sinus arrhythmia

    C.   Sinus bradycardia

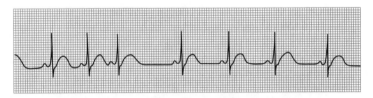

17. A 45-year-old patient is admitted with an acute MI. In the emergency department, he received nitroglycerin and morphine to treat his chest pain, and he's currently pain-free. His monitor reveals sinus tachycardia at a rate of 123 beats/minute. Which statement is true regarding sinus tachycardia after acute MI?

    A.   Sinus tachycardia is a normal response that typically abates after the first 24 hours.

    B.   Sinus tachycardia is a poor prognostic sign because it may be associated with massive heart damage.

    C.   Sinus tachycardia is a typical response to morphine administration.

18. An 83-year-old patient is admitted from a long-term care facility with severe dehydration. You begin cardiac monitoring and record the rhythm strip shown below. What are the strip's characteristics?

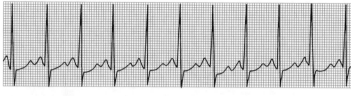

Atrial rhythm: _____   QRS complex:_____
Ventricular rhythm: _____   T wave: _____
Atrial rate: _____   QT interval:_____
Ventricular rate: _____   Other: _____
P wave: _____   Interpretation: _____
PR interval:_____   _____

19. A patient is admitted to your telemetry unit with a diagnosis of sick sinus syndrome. Which medication should you keep readily available to treat a symptomatic event?
    A.   isoproterenol (Isuprel)
    B.   verapamil (Calan)
    C.   atropine

20. A patient develops sinus bradycardia. Which symptoms indicate that his cardiac output is falling?
    A.   Hypertension and further drop in heart rate
    B.   Hypotension and dizziness
    C.   Increased urine output and syncope

21. A patient admitted 2 days ago with an acute MI suddenly develops premature atrial contractions. What's the most likely cause of this arrhythmia in this patient?
    A.   Increased caffeine intake
    B.   Impending cardiogenic shock
    C.   Developing heart failure

22. A patient admitted with an exacerbation of chronic obstructive pulmonary disease is being monitored. At the beginning of your shift, you print out the following rhythm strip. What's your interpretation of this strip?

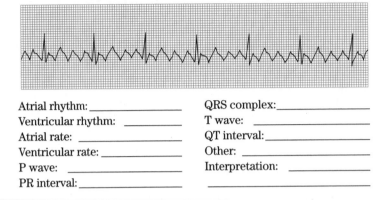

Atrial rhythm: _____   QRS complex: _____

Ventricular rhythm: _____   T wave: _____

Atrial rate: _____   QT interval: _____

Ventricular rate: _____   Other: _____

P wave: _____   Interpretation: _____

PR interval: _____   _____

23. You're caring for a patient with digoxin toxicity who develops the following rhythm. You print a strip and analyze it. What's your interpretation of the strip?

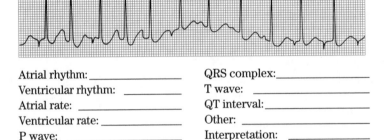

Atrial rhythm: _____   QRS complex: _____

Ventricular rhythm: _____   T wave: _____

Atrial rate: _____   QT interval: _____

Ventricular rate: _____   Other: _____

P wave: _____   Interpretation: _____

PR interval: _____   _____

24. A patient diagnosed with heart failure is admitted to your telemetry unit. She complains of seeing yellow-green halos around visual images. She also states that she's been nauseous and unable to eat for the past few days. Based on these findings you suspect:

    A.   digoxin toxicity.

    B.   atrial fibrillation.

    C.   worsening heart failure.

25. A patient returns to your unit after cardiac surgery. As you perform your assessment of the patient, you note that his cardiac monitor show atrial fibrillation at a rate of 160 beats/minute. The patient suddenly begins complaining of chest pain. Based on these findings, what's the best treatment?

    A.   digoxin administration

    B.   Defibrillation

    C.   Cardioversion

26. A 32-year-old patient with a history of Wolff-Parkinson-White syndrome is admitted to your floor following gallbladder surgery. Which of the following ECG characteristics are typical in a patient with Wolff-Parkinson-White syndrome?

    A.   Prolonged PR interval and narrow QRS complex

    B.   Prolonged PR interval and presence of a delta wave

    C.   Widened QRS complex and presence of a delta wave

27. A 68-year-old patient with a history of heart failure is receiving digoxin. At the beginning of your shift you record the patient's rhythm strip shown below. You interpret this rhythm as:

    A.   junctional tachycardia.

    B.   wandering pacemaker.

    C.   accelerated junctional rhythm.

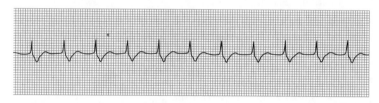

28. A 54-year-old patient is admitted to your unit with an acute MI. While you're assessing the patient, he tells you that his heart keeps skipping a beat. You record the strip below from his cardiac monitor. What are the strip's characteristics?

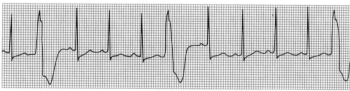

Atrial rhythm: _____   QRS complex:_____

Ventricular rhythm: _____   T wave: _____

Atrial rate: _____   QT interval:_____

Ventricular rate: _____   Other: _____

P wave: _____   Interpretation: _____

PR interval:_____   _____

29. A patient with a history of chronic obstructive pulmonary disease is admitted to your floor with hypoxemia. You begin cardiac monitoring, which reveals the rhythm shown below. You interpret this rhythm as:

    A.   premature junctional contractions.
    B.   wandering pacemaker.
    C.   accelerated junctional rhythm.

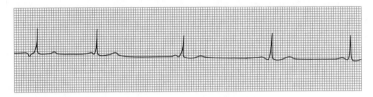

30. A patient is admitted to your unit with digoxin toxicity. You record a rhythm strip and note that the rhythm is regular, rate is 80 beats/minute, and P waves are inverted in lead II and occur before each QRS complex. Based on these findings you interpret the rhythm as:

    A.   accelerated junctional rhythm.
    B.   junctional tachycardia.
    C.   junctional escape rhythm.

31. A patient with an acute MI develops the arrhythmia below. He's asymptomatic. You record the rhythm strip and identify the arrhythmia as:

    A.   idioventricular rhythm.
    B.   junctional escape rhythm.
    C.   premature junctional contraction.

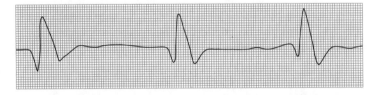

32. A patient with the arrhythmia identified above suddenly becomes hypotensive. You must immediately administer which agent to increase his heart rate?

    A.   lidocaine
    B.   isoproterenol
    C.   atropine

33. A 78-year-old patient is admitted to your floor with dehydration after dosing herself with extra furosemide. Her admission potassium is 2.5 mEq/L. You're administering a potassium supplement when you notice the following rhythm on her cardiac monitor. What's your interpretation of this strip?

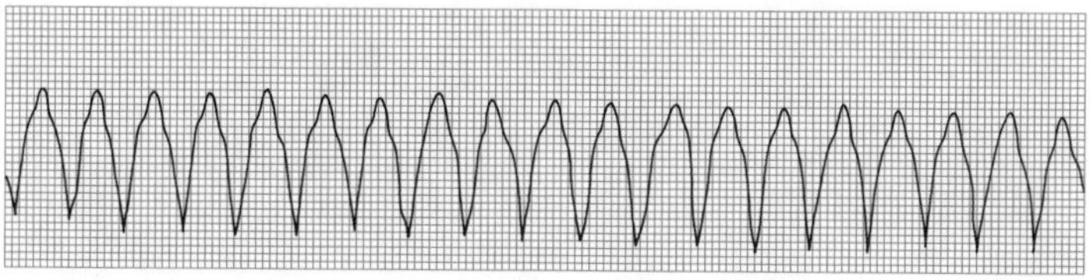

Atrial rhythm: _____   QRS complex:_____

Ventricular rhythm: _____   T wave: _____

Atrial rate: _____   QT interval:_____

Ventricular rate:_____   Other: _____

P wave: _____   Interpretation: _____

PR interval:_____   _____

34. You deliver synchronized cardioversion to a patient with monomorphic ventricular tachycardia. The monitor suddenly displays the following rhythm. What's your interpretation?

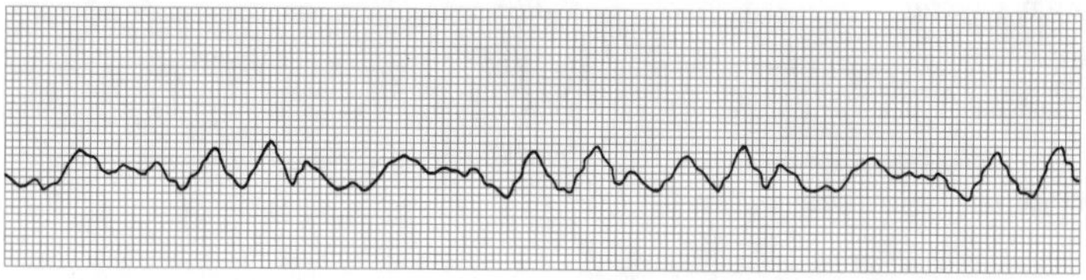

Atrial rhythm: _____   QRS complex:_____

Ventricular rhythm: _____   T wave: _____

Atrial rate: _____   QT interval:_____

Ventricular rate:_____   Other: _____

P wave: _____   Interpretation: _____

PR interval:_____   _____

35. A patient with a low magnesium level develops the following arrhythmia. You interpret the rhythm as:

A.   monomorphic ventricular tachycardia.

B.   ventricular fibrillation

C.   torsades de pointes.

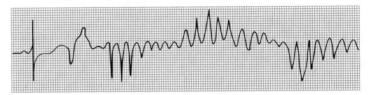

36. Following cardiac surgery, your patient's cardiac monitor displays the following rhythm strip. How would you interpret the strip?

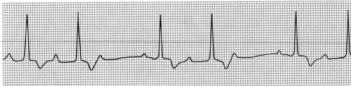

Atrial rhythm: _____   QRS complex:_____

Ventricular rhythm: _____   T wave: _____

Atrial rate: _____   QT interval:_____

Ventricular rate: _____   Other: _____

P wave: _____   Interpretation: _____

PR interval:_____   _____

37. An 83-year-old patient is brought to the emergency department after her daughter reported that the patient took an accidental overdose of her calcium channel blocker. After you begin cardiac monitoring, you record the following rhythm strip. What's your interpretation of the strip?

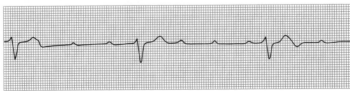

Atrial rhythm: _____   QRS complex:_____

Ventricular rhythm: _____   T wave: _____

Atrial rate: _____   QT interval:_____

Ventricular rate: _____   Other: _____

P wave: _____   Interpretation: _____

PR interval:_____   _____

38. A patient with an acute anterior wall MI develops third-degree heart block. His blood pressure is 78/44 mm Hg, and he's complaining of dizziness. You should immediately administer atropine and:

    A.   administer isoproterenol.

    B.   apply a transcutaneous pacemaker.

    C.   place the patient in Trendelenburg's position.

39. An 86-year-old patient is found in her apartment without heat on a cold winter day. She's admitted to your unit with hypothermia. You begin cardiac monitoring, which displays the rhythm shown below. You document this strip as:

    A.   first-degree AV block.

    B.   sinus tachycardia.

    C.   junctional tachycardia.

40. A patient is receiving quinidine for treatment of atrial fibrillation. You record a rhythm strip at the beginning of your shift. How would you interpret the strip?

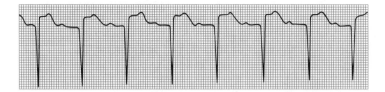

Atrial rhythm: _____   QRS complex: _____

Ventricular rhythm: _____   T wave: _____

Atrial rate: _____   QT interval: _____

Ventricular rate: _____   Other: _____

P wave: _____   Interpretation: _____

PR interval: _____   _____

41. You're caring for a patient who developed complications after an acute MI requiring transcutaneous pacemaker insertion. His monitor alarm sounds and the following rhythm strip is recorded. You recognize this as which type of pacemaker malfunction?

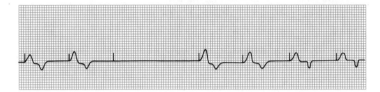

    A.   Failure to capture
    B.   Failure to pace
    C.   Failure to sense

42. A patient admitted to the cardiac care unit with digoxin toxicity required transcutaneous pacemaker insertion. While assessing the patient, you note the following rhythm on the patient's monitor. This rhythm strip displays:
    A.   oversensing.
    B.   failure to sense.
    C.   failure to pace.

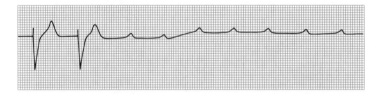

43. Your patient signals you to come into his room. As you approach his bedside, he complains that his heart is skipping beats. You immediately record a rhythm strip from his cardiac monitor and take his vital signs. Based on the recorded rhythm strip, you should notify the doctor of:
    A.   failure to sense.
    B.   oversensing.
    C.   pacemaker-mediated tachycardia.

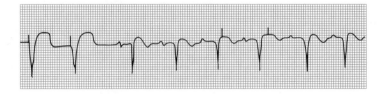

44. A 54-year-old patient returns to your telemetry unit after permanent pacemaker insertion for sick sinus syndrome. When you record a rhythm strip, you note that the pacemaker is malfunctioning. You document your finding as:

    A.   failure to sense.

    B.   failure to pace.

    C.   oversensing.

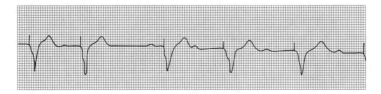

45. When developing a teaching plan for the patient with a newly inserted permanent pacemaker, you should include:

    A.   advising the patient to avoid computed tomography scans.

    B.   telling the patient that hiccups are normal for the first few days after pacemaker insertion.

    C.   instructing the patient to avoid tight clothing.

46. You're caring for a 75-year-old patient who's prescribed oral procainamide to control a supraventricular tachycardia. Before discharge you should instruct the patient:

    A.   to avoid chewing the drug, which may cause him to get too much of the drug at once.

    B.   that lupus-like symptoms are normal and will cease in 2 to 3 weeks after initiation of therapy

    C.   that a bitter taste is common.

47. A patient returns to your floor from the postanesthesia care unit after undergoing a right lower lobectomy. When you begin cardiac monitoring, you note the following rhythm strip. Which drug will the doctor most likely prescribe to rapidly convert this rhythm?

    A.   propafenone

    B.   tocainide

    C.   ibutilide

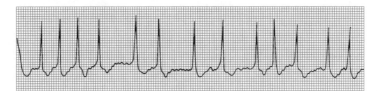

48. After receiving quinidine, you note that your patient's QT interval is prolonged on his rhythm strip. You notify the doctor immediately because you know that prolongation of the QT interval places the patient at risk for what?

    A.   Atrial fibrillation

    B.   Junctional tachycardia

    C.   Polymorphic ventricular tachycardia

49. A 74-year-old patient is admitted to your floor from the emergency department with syncope. You note the following rhythm when you record a rhythm strip from his cardiac monitor. Based on this rhythm strip, you should question an order for which drug on the patient's chart?

    A.   bretylium

    B.   verapamil

    C.   epinephrine

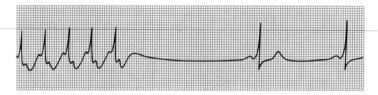

50. A 36-year-old patient with a history of heart transplantation is admitted to your floor for observation after an appendectomy. If the patient develops symptomatic bradycardia, which drug is indicated?

    A.   atropine

    B.   isoproterenol

    C.   dopamine

51. The doctor orders a preoperative 12-lead ECG for your patient who's scheduled for a thoracotomy in the morning. Using your knowledge of 12-lead ECGs, which leads are bipolar?

    A. aV_R, aV_L, and aV_F

    B.   I, II, and III

    C. V_1, V_2, and V_3

52. Each of the 12 leads of an ECG views the heart from a different angle. Lead I views which area of the heart?

    A.   Inferior wall

    B.   Anterior wall

    C.   Lateral wall

53. You're caring for a patient with a history of angina who calls you into his room because he's experiencing chest pain. His admission orders included a 12-lead ECG with each episode of chest pain. You immediately retrieve the ECG machine. To ensure proper placement, where should you place lead V_1?

    A.   Over the fourth intercostal space at the right sternal border

    B.   Over the fourth intercostal space at the left sternal border

    C.   Over the fifth intercostal space at the left anterior axillary line

54. A patient, who sustained an acute MI, is ordered a signal-averaged ECG. Why is this test typically ordered?

    A.   To locate posterior wall damage

    B.   To identify whether the patient is at risk for sudden death from sustained ventricular tachycardia

    C.   To identify whether the patient has suffered damage to his right ventricle

55. A 12-lead ECG is ordered for a 32-year-old patient who comes to the emergency department complaining of chest pain. You know that a 12-lead ECG is necessary to assess function of the:

    A.   right ventricle.

    B.   right and left ventricles.

    C.   left ventricle.

56. You're caring for a 72-year-old patient admitted with unstable angina. He calls you into his room and complains of chest pain that he rates an 8 on a scale of 1 to 10 (10 being the worst). You immediately obtain a 12-lead ECG. Which ECG change would you expect with angina?

    A.   Pathologic Q wave

    B.   T-wave inversion

    C.   Widened QRS complex

57. A patient's 12-lead ECG reveals left axis deviation. When is left axis deviation considered normal?

    A.   In infants

    B.   In small children

    C.   In pregnant women

58. A 38-year-old patient is admitted with a diagnosis of unstable angina. Which statement is true about unstable angina?

    A.   The pain is typically triggered by exertion or stress.

    B.   The pain is typically relieved by rest.

    C.   The pain may occur while the patient is sleeping.

59. After experiencing substernal chest pain for about 4 hours, a patient drives himself to the emergency department. He is triaged immediately and a 12-lead ECG is obtained. Which change on the patient's ECG is associated with myocardial necrosis?

A.   Pathologic Q waves

B.   T-wave inversion

C.   ST-segment elevation

60. When examining your patient's 12-lead ECG, you notice a bundle-branch block. Which leads should you check to determine whether the block is in the right or left bundle?

A. V_1 and V_6

B.   II and aV_F

C. V_4 and V_5

Answers

1. A. The bicuspid valve, commonly called the mitral valve is located between the left atrium and left ventricle.

2. B. The circumflex artery supplies oxygenated blood to the lateral walls of the ventricle, the left atrium, and to the left posterior fasciculus of the left bundle branch.

3. B. The vagus nerve carries impulses that slow the heart rate and the conduction of impulses through the AV node and ventricles.

4. B. Polarization describes cardiac cells at rest.

5. C. If the Purkinje fibers take over as the heart's pacemaker, impulses are typically discharged at a rate of 20 to 40 times per minute.

6. A. The six limb leads — leads I, II, III, aV_R, aV_L, and aV_F — provide information about the heart's frontal plane.

7. C. V_1 on a 12-lead ECG is the equivalent to MCL_1.

8. A. Before initiating cardiac monitoring, you must first prepare the patient's skin. Use a special rough patch on the back of the electrode, a dry washcloth, or a gauze pad to briskly rub each site until the skin reddens.

9. A. Electrical interference appears on the ECG as a baseline that's thick and unreadable. Electrical interference is caused by electrical power leakage. It may also occur due to interference from other equipment in the room or improperly grounded equipment.

10. B. The horizontal axis of the ECG strip represents time.

11. C. Using the 8-step method of rhythm strip interpretation, you should check the rhythm first and then calculate the rate. Next, evaluate the P wave, check out the PR interval and the QRS complex, examine the T wave, measure the QT interval and, finally, check for ectopic beats and other abnormalities.

12. B. A change in the ST segment may indicate myocardial damage. An ST segment may become either elevated or depressed.

13. A. A U wave isn't present on every rhythm strip. A prominent U wave may be due to hypokalemia, hypercalcemia, or digoxin toxicity.

14. A. You can use the 10-times method, the 1,500 method, or the sequence method to determine heart rate. However, don't rely on these methods. Always check a pulse to correlate it with the heart rate on the ECG.

15. B. The normal duration of a PR interval is 0.12 to 0.20 second.

16. B. The rhythm strip shows sinus arrhythmia. If sinus arrhythmia develops suddenly in the patient taking digoxin, the patient may be experiencing digoxin toxicity.

17. B. Sinus tachycardia occurs in about 30% of patients after acute MI and is considered a poor prognostic sign because it may be associated with massive heart damage.

18. Rhythm: both regular
Rate: both — 110 beats/minute
P wave: normal size and configuration
PR interval: 0.16 second
QRS complex: 0.10 second
T wave: normal configuration
QT interval: 0.36 second
Other: none
Interpretation: sinus tachycardia

19. C. Atropine or epinephrine may be administered for a symptomatic acute attack. Therefore, you should keep these drugs readily available.

20. B. When sinus bradycardia is symptomatic, the resulting drop in cardiac output produces such signs and symptoms as hypotension and dizziness.

21. C. In a patient with an acute MI, PACs can serve as an early sign of heart failure or an electrolyte imbalance.

22. Rhythm: both regular
Rate: Atrial — 270 beats/minute; ventricular — 70 beats/minute
P wave: saw-tooth edged
PR interval: immeasurable
QRS complex: 0.10 second
T wave: unidentifiable
QT interval: unidentifiable
Other: none
Interpretation: atrial flutter (4:1 block)

23. Rhythm: both irregular
Rate: about 150 beats/minute
P wave: three types of P waves are seen
PR interval: varies
QRS complex: 0.08 second
T wave: inverted
QT interval: 0.22 second
Other: none
Interpretation: multifocal atrial tachycardia

24. A. The patient with digoxin toxicity may develop arrhythmias, blurred vision, hypotension, increased severity of heart failure, yellow-green halos around visual images, anorexia, nausea, and vomiting.

25. C. If the patient with atrial fibrillation complains of chest pain, emergency measures such as cardioversion are necessary. Digoxin may be used to control the ventricular response in patients with atrial fibrillation who are asymptomatic.

26. C. Wolff-Parkinson-White syndrome causes a shortened PR interval (less than 0.10 second) and a widened QRS complex (greater than 0.10 second). The beginning of the QRS complex may appear slurred. This hallmark sign is referred to as a delta wave.

27. A. A rhythm strip reveals junctional tachycardia. The rhythm is regular, rate 110 beats/minute, a P wave occurs after each QRS complex, and the PR interval is immeasurable.

28. Rhythm: both irregular
Rate: both — 105 beats/minute
P wave: normal size and configuration except during premature beat
PR interval: 0.16 second; immeasurable for premature beat
QRS complex: 0.06 second
T wave: normal configuration
QT interval: 0.36 second
Other: none
Interpretation: sinus tachycardia with premature ventricular contractions

29. B. The rhythm strip reveals a wandering pacemaker. The key characteristics are the varying shapes of the P waves.

30. A. Based on these findings, the patient's rhythm strip reveals accelerated junctional rhythm.

31. A. The rhythm strip reveals idioventricular rhythm.

32. C. The agent of choice for treatment of idioventricular rhythm is atropine. A pacemaker may be necessary after atropine administration.

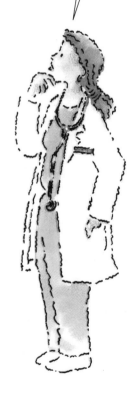

A slurred QRS complex is referred to as a delta wave.

33. Rhythm: atrial — can't be determined; ventricular — regular
Rate: atrial — can't be determined; ventricular — 187 beats/minute
P wave: absent
PR interval: immeasurable
QRS complex: 0.18 second; wide and bizarre
T wave: opposite direction of QRS complex
QT interval: immeasurable
Other: none
Interpretation: ventricular tachycardia (monomorphic)

34. Rhythm: atrial — immeasurable; ventricular — immeasurable, fibrillatory waves present
Rate: immeasurable
P wave: absent
PR interval: none
QRS complex: immeasurable
T wave: opposite direction of QRS complex
QT interval: none
Other: none
Interpretation: ventricular fibrillation

35. C. The strip shows torsades de pointes.

36. Rhythm: atrial — regular; ventricular — irregular
Rate: atrial — 75 beats/minute; ventricular — 50 beats/minute
P wave: normal size and configuration
PR interval: lengthens with each cycle until dropped
QRS complex: 0.06 second
T wave: normal configuration
QT interval: 0.38 second
Other: none
Interpretation: type I (Mobitz I or Wenckebach) second-degree AV block

37. Rhythm: atrial — regular; ventricular — regular
Rate: atrial — 90 beats/minute; ventricular — 30 beats/minute
P wave: normal size and configuration except when hidden within the T wave
PR interval: varies
QRS complex: 0.16 second
T wave: normal configuration
QT interval: 0.56 second
Other: none
Interpretation: third-degree AV block

38. B. If the patient's cardiac output is inadequate (low blood pressure and dizziness), you should immediately administer atropine and apply a transcutaneous pacemaker. The patient may need a temporary pacemaker until the block resolves. If the patient has permanent heart block, he'll need a permanent pacemaker.

39. A. You should document in your notes that the patient's monitor reveals a first-degree atrioventricular block. Hypothermia is one cause of this arrhythmia.

40. Rhythm: atrial — regular; ventricular — regular
Rate: atrial and ventricular — 60 beats/minute
P wave: normal size and configuration
PR interval: 0.36 second
QRS complex: 0.08 second
T wave: normal configuration
QT interval: 0.40 second
Other: none
Interpretation: first-degree AV block

41. A. The rhythm strip shows the pacemaker's failure to capture. The ECG pacemaker spike isn't followed by a QRS complex.

42. C. The rhythm strip reveals the pacemaker's failure to pace. After two paced beats there's no apparent pacemaker activity on the ECG.

43. A. The ECG pacemaker spikes fall where they shouldn't, indicating a failure to sense.

44. C. You document that the pacemaker is oversensing and report the finding to the doctor immediately. Reprogramming of the pacemaker may be necessary.

45. C. You should instruct the patient to avoid tight clothing or any direct pressure over the pulse generator, to avoid magnetic resonance imaging scans and certain other diagnostic studies, and to notify the doctor if he feels confused, light-headed, or short of breath. The patient should also notify the doctor if he has palpitations, hiccups, or a rapid or unusually slow heart rate.

46. C. Warn the patient taking procainamide orally not to chew it, which might cause him to get too much of the drug at once. Lupus-like symptoms are associated with long-term use of procainamide and may require discontinuation of the drug. A bitter taste is also an adverse effect of procainamide.

47. C. This rhythm strip reveals atrial fibrillation. Ibutilide is used for rapid conversion of recent-onset atrial fibrillation or flutter to sinus rhythm.

48. C. Prolongation of the QT interval is a sign that the patient is predisposed to developing polymorphic ventricular tachycardia.

49. B. The rhythm strip reveals sick sinus syndrome. Verapamil should be avoided in sick sinus syndrome or second- or third-degree AV block without a pacemaker and in atrial fibrillation or flutter due to Wolff-Parkinson-White syndrome.

50. B. Isoproterenol is the drug of choice for treating symptomatic bradycardia in patients who have undergone heart transplantation. The vagal nerve dissection that occurs during heart transplantation surgery renders atropine ineffective in these patients.

51. B. The 12 leads include three bipolar limb leads (I, II, and III), three unipolar augmented limb leads (aV_R, aV_L, and aV_F) and six unipolar precordial leads (V_1, V_2, V_3, V_4, V_5, and V_6).

52. C. Lead I views the lateral wall of the heart.

53. A. Lead V_1 should be placed over the fourth intercostal space at the right sternal border.

54. B. Signal-averaged ECG helps identify patients at risk for sudden death from sustained ventricular tachycardia. The test uses a computer to identify late electrical potentials that can't be detected by a 12-lead ECG.

55. C. A 12-lead ECG is used to assess left ventricular function. A right-sided ECG is necessary to assess right ventricular function.

56. B. Classic ECG changes associated with angina include peaked T wave, flattened T wave, T-wave inversion, ST-segment depression with T-wave inversion, and ST-segment depression without T-wave inversion.

57. C. Left axis deviation is a normal finding in pregnant women. Right axis deviation is normal in infants and small children.

58. C. In stable angina, pain is triggered by exertion or stress and is commonly relieved by rest. Each episode follows a similar pattern. Unstable angina is more easily provoked and may occur while the patient is sleeping, causing him to awaken. It's also unpredictable and tends to worsen over time.

59. A. The area of myocardial necrosis is called the zone of infarction. The ECG change associated with a necrotic area is a pathologic Q wave. The zone of injury shows up on an ECG as an elevated ST segment. The zone of ischemia is represented by T-wave inversion.

60. A. After you identify a bundle-branch block, examine lead V_1, which lies to the right of the heart, and lead V_6, which lies to the left of the heart. These leads will tell you if the block is in the right or left bundle.

Quick guide to arrhythmias

Use this chart as a quick reference for identifying characteristics of cardiac arrhythmias. Here are the characteristics of a normal rhythm strip.
- Atrial and ventricular rates are 60 to 100 beats/minute
- Atrial and ventricular rhythms are regular
- PR interval is 0.12 to 0.2 second
- QRS duration is less than 0.12 second
- QT interval is 0.36 to 0.44 second

Arrhythmia and features	Causes	Treatment
Sinus arrhythmia • Irregular atrial and ventricular rhythms; corresponds with respiratory cycle • Normal P wave preceding each QRS complex	• A normal variation of sinus rhythm in athletes, children, and older adults • Also seen with digoxin use, morphine use, increased intracranial pressure (ICP), and inferior wall myocardial infarction (MI)	• Typically no treatment is necessary; may correct underlying cause
Sinus tachycardia • Atrial and ventricular rhythms regular • Atrial and ventricular rates are equal; generally 100 to 160 beats/minute • Normal P wave preceding each QRS complex	• Normal physiologic response to fever, exercise, stress, fear, anxiety, pain, dehydration; may also accompany shock, left-sided heart failure, pericarditis, hyperthyroidism, anemia, pulmonary embolism, or sepsis • May also occur with atropine, isoproterenol, aminophylline, dopamine, dobutamine, epinephrine, quinidine, caffeine, alcohol, amphetamine, or nicotine use	• No treatment is necessary if patient is asymptomatic • Correction of underlying cause
Sinus bradycardia • Regular atrial and ventricular rhythms • Rate less than 60 beats/minute • Normal P wave preceding each QRS complex	• Normal during sleep and in well-conditioned heart such as in an athlete • Increased ICP; Valsalva's maneuver, carotid sinus massage, vomiting, hypothyroidism; hyperkalemia, hypothermia, cardiomyopathy, or inferior wall MI • May also occur with beta blockers, calcium channel blockers, lithium, sotalol, amiodarone, digoxin, or quinidine use	• No treatment necessary if patient is asymptomatic; if drugs are the cause, may need to discontinue use • For low cardiac output, dizziness, weakness, altered level of consciousness, or low blood pressure: 0.5 to 1.0 mg atropine • Temporary pacemaker or permanent pacemaker if condition becomes chronic

Arrhythmia and features	Causes	Treatment
Sinus arrest • Atrial and ventricular rhythms normal except for missing complex • Normal P wave preceding each QRS complex	• Coronary artery disease (CAD), acute myocarditis, or acute inferior wall MI • Increased vagal tone as occurs with Valsalva's maneuver, carotid sinus massage, or vomiting • Digoxin, quinidine, procainamide and salicylates, especially if given at toxic levels • Excessive doses of beta blockers, such as metoprolol and propranolol • Sinus node disease	• No treatment necessary if patient is asymptomatic • For mild symptoms, may stop medications that contribute to arrhythmia • If symptomatic, administer atropine • Temporary or permanent pacemaker for repeated episodes
Premature atrial contractions (PACs) • Premature, abnormal-looking P waves, differing in configuration from normal P waves • QRS complexes after P waves, except in blocked PACs • P wave often buried in the preceding T wave or identified in the preceding T wave	• Triggered by alcohol, cigarettes, anxiety, fever, and infectious disease in a normal heart • Heart failure, coronary or valvular heart disease, acute respiratory failure, chronic obstructive pulmonary disease (COPD), electrolyte imbalance, or hypoxia • Digoxin toxicity	• No treatment necessary if patient is asymptomatic • If frequent, may treat with digoxin, procainamide, or verapamil • Treatment of underlying cause; patient may need to avoid caffeine or smoking and learn stress reduction measures
Atrial tachycardia • Atrial and ventricular rhythms regular when block is constant; irregular when it isn't • Heart rate 150 to 250 beats/minute • P waves regular but hidden in preceding T wave; precede QRS complexes • Sudden onset and termination of arrhythmia	• Physical or psychological stress, hypoxia, electrolyte imbalances, cardiomyopathy, congenital anomalies, MI, valvular disease, Wolff-Parkinson-White syndrome, cor pulmonale, hyperthyroidism, or systemic hypertension • Digoxin toxicity; caffeine, marijuana, or stimulant use	• Vagal stimulation, Valsalva's maneuver, and carotid sinus massage • Treatment priority is decreasing the ventricular response by using a calcium-channel blocker, beta-adrenergic blocker, digoxin, and cardioversion; then consider procainamide or amiodarone, if each preceding treatment is ineffective in rhythm conversion • If the ejection fraction is less than 40% or the patient is in heart failure, treat with cardioversion or amiodarone

Arrhythmia and features	Causes	Treatment
Atrial flutter • Atrial rhythm regular; rate is 250 to 400 beats/minute • Ventricular rhythm variable, depending on degree of atrioventricular (AV) block; rate usually 60 to 100 beats/minute • Sawtooth P-wave configuration possible (F waves) • QRS complexes uniform in shape but often irregular in rate	• Heart failure, severe mitral valve disease, hyperthyroidism, pericardial disease, COPD, systemic arterial hypoxia, and acute MI	• Treatment of underlying cause • Synchronized cardioversion is the treatment of choice • Drug therapy includes digoxin and calcium channel blockers • Ibutilide fumarate may be used to convert recent-onset atrial flutter to sinus rhythm
Atrial fibrillation • Atrial rhythm grossly irregular; atrial rate greater than 400 beats/minute • Ventricular rhythm grossly irregular • QRS complexes of uniform configuration and duration • PR interval indiscernible • No P waves; replaced by fine fibrillatory waves	• Inferior wall MI, hypoxia, vagal stimulation, or sick sinus syndrome • Rheumatic heart disease • Digoxin toxicity	• Control ventricular response with drugs such as diltiazem, verapamil, digoxin, and beta-adrenergic blockers. • Ibutilide fumarate may be used to convert new-onset atrial fibrillation to sinus rhythm • Quinidine and procainamide can also convert atrial fibrillation to normal sinus rhythm, usually after anticoagulation • Synchronized cardioversion is most successful if used within the first 3 days of treatment
Junctional escape rhythm • Atrial and ventricular rhythms regular • Atrial rate 40 to 60 beats/minute • Ventricular rate 40 to 60 beats/minute (60 to 100 beats/minute is accelerated junctional rhythm) • P waves before, hidden in, or after QRS complex; inverted, if visible • PR interval is less than 0.12 second and is measurable only if the P wave comes before the QRS complex • QRS complex configuration and duration normal	• Inferior wall MI, rheumatic heart disease, valvular disease, swelling of the AV junction after heart surgery • Digoxin toxicity and excessive caffeine use	• Atropine for symptomatic slow rate • Pacemaker insertion, if refractory to drugs • Discontinuation of digoxin, if appropriate

Arrhythmia and features	Causes	Treatment
Premature junctional contractions • Atrial and ventricular rhythms irregular • P waves inverted; may precede, be hidden within, or follow QRS complex • PR interval less than 0.12 second, if P wave precedes QRS complex • QRS complex configuration and duration normal	• Inferior- or posterior-wall MI or ischemia, congenital heart disease in children, swelling of the AV junction after surgery • Digoxin toxicity (most common)	• Correction of underlying cause • Discontinuation of digoxin, if appropriate • May require elimination of caffeine intake
Junctional tachycardia • Atrial rate is 100 to 200 beats/minute; however, P wave may be absent, be hidden in QRS complex, or precede T wave • Ventricular rate is 100 to 200 beats/minute • P wave inverted • QRS complex configuration and duration normal	• Rheumatic carditis as a result of inflammation involving the SA node • Digoxin toxicity • Sick sinus syndrome	• Correction of the underlying cause • Discontinuation of digoxin, if appropriate • Pacemaker insertion may be necessary
Wandering pacemaker • Atrial and ventricular rhythms are irregular • PR interval varies • P waves change in configuration indicating that impulses may originate in the sinoatrial (SA) node, atria, or AV junction	• May be normal in young patients, and is common in athletes who have slow heart rates • Rheumatic carditis, increased vagal tone • Digoxin toxicity	• No treatment if patient is asymptomatic • Treatment of underlying cause if patient is symptomatic
First-degree AV block • Atrial and ventricular rhythms regular • PR interval greater than 0.20 second • P wave preceding each QRS complex; QRS complex normal	• May be seen in a healthy person • Myocardial ischemia or infarction, myocarditis, or degenerative heart changes • Digoxin, calcium channel blocker, and beta blocker use	• Cautious use of digoxin • Correction of underlying cause

Arrhythmia and features	Causes	Treatment
Type I second-degree AV block Mobitz I (Wenckebach) • Atrial rhythm regular • Ventricular rhythm irregular • Atrial rate exceeds ventricular rate • PR interval progressively, but only slightly, longer with each cycle until QRS complex disappears (dropped beat)	• Inferior wall MI, CAD, rheumatic fever, or vagal stimulation • Digoxin toxicity; propranolol or verapamil use	• Treatment of underlying cause • Atropine or temporary pacemaker for symptomatic bradycardia • Discontinuation of digoxin, if appropriate
Type II second-degree AV block Mobitz II • Atrial rhythm regular • Ventricular rhythm regular or irregular, with varying degree of block • QRS complexes periodically absent	• Severe CAD, anterior MI, or degenerative changes in the conduction system • Digoxin toxicity	• Atropine for symptomatic bradycardia • Temporary pacemaker • Discontinuation of digoxin, if appropriate
Third-degree AV block (complete heart block) • Atrial rhythm regular • Ventricular rhythm slow and regular; if escape rhythm originates in the AV node the rate is 40 to 60 beats/minute, if escape rhythm originates in the Purkinje system the rate is less than 40 beats/minute • No relation between P waves and QRS complexes • PR interval can't be measured • QRS interval normal (originates in the AV node) or wide and bizarre (originates in the Purkinje system)	• Inferior or anterior wall MI, CAD, degenerative changes in the heart, congenital abnormality, hypoxia, surgical injury • Digoxin toxicity	• Atropine for symptomatic bradycardia • Temporary or permanent pacemaker

Arrhythmia and features	Causes	Treatment
Premature ventricular contractions (PVCs) • Atrial rate regular in underlying rhythm; P wave is absent with premature beat • Ventricular rate irregular during PVC; underlying rhythm may be regular • QRS complex premature, usually followed by a complete compensatory pause • QRS complex wide and bizarre, usually greater than 0.12 second in the premature beat • Premature QRS complexes occurring singly, in pairs, or in threes; alternating with normal beats; focus from one or more sites • Most ominous when clustered, multifocal, with R wave on T pattern	• Heart failure; myocardial ischemia, infarction, or contusion; myocarditis, myocardial irritation by ventricular catheter such as a pacemaker; hypokalemia metabolic acidosis; or hypocalcemia • Drug intoxication, particularly with cocaine, tricyclic antidepressants, and amphetamines • Caffeine, tobacco, or alcohol use • Psychological stress; anxiety; pain; or exercise	• If symptomatic, administer procainamide • Treatment of underlying cause • Discontinuation of drug causing toxicity • Potassium chloride I.V. if induced by hypokalemia
Ventricular tachycardia • Ventricular rate 100 to 200 beats/minute; rhythm is regular or irregular • QRS complexes wide, bizarre, and independent of P waves; duration is greater than 0.12 second • P waves not discernible • May start and stop suddenly	• Myocardial ischemia, or infarction, CAD; valvular heart disease; heart failure; cardiomyopathy; ventricular catheters; hypokalemia; hypercalcemia; or pulmonary embolism • Digoxin, procainamide, quinidine, or cocaine toxicity • Anxiety	• If patient is pulseless, immediate cardioversion and resuscitation • If monomorphic ventricular tachycardia, procainamide is given to try to correct the rhythm disturbance; then other drugs such as amiodarone are used • If polymorphic ventricular tachycardia, a beta-adrenergic blocker, amiodarone, or procainamide may be given • If patient develops recurrent episodes of ventricular tachycardia unresponsive to drug therapy, a cardioverter-defibrillator may be implanted

Arrhythmia and features	Causes	Treatment
Ventricular fibrillation • Ventricular rhythm rapid and chaotic • QRS complexes wide and irregular; no visible P waves	• Myocardial ischemia or infarction, untreated ventricular tachycardia, hypokalemia, acid-base imbalances, hyperkalemia, hypercalcemia, electric shock, or severe hypothermia • Digoxin, epinephrine, or quinidine toxicity	• Rapid defibrillation • Epinephrine or vasopressin followed by defibrillation • Consider antiarrhythmics such as amiodarone or magnesium • Cardiopulmonary resuscitation (CPR) • Treatment of underlying cause
Asystole • No atrial or ventricular rate or rhythm • No discernible P waves, QRS complexes, or T waves	• Myocardial ischemia or infarction, heart failure, prolonged hypoxemia, severe electrolyte disturbances such as hyperkalemia, severe acid-base disturbances, electric shock, ventricular arrhythmias, atrioventricular block, pulmonary embolism, or cardiac tamponade • Cocaine overdose	• CPR, following advanced cardiac life-support protocol • Endotracheal intubation • Transcutaneous pacemaker • Treatment of underlying cause • Repeated doses of epinephrine, as ordered

Glossary

aberrant conduction: abnormal pathway of an impulse traveling through the heart's conduction system

ablation: surgical or radio-frequency removal of an irritable focus in the heart; used to prevent tachyarrhythmias

afterload: resistance that the left ventricle must work against to pump blood through the aorta

amplitude: height of a waveform

arrhythmia: disturbance of the normal cardiac rhythm from the abnormal origin, discharge, or conduction of electrical impulses

artifact: waveforms in an ECG tracing that don't originate in the heart

atrial kick: amount of blood pumped into the ventricles as a result of atrial contraction; contributes approximately 30% of total cardiac output

automaticity: ability of a cardiac cell to initiate an impulse on its own

bigeminy: premature beat occurring every other beat; alternates with normal QRS complexes

biotransformation: series of chemical changes of a substance as a result of enzyme activity; end result of drug biotransformation may be active or inactive metabolites

biphasic: complex containing both an upward and a downward deflection; usually seen when the electrical current is perpendicular to the observed lead

bundle-branch block: slowing or blocking of an impulse as it travels through one of the bundle branches

capture: successful pacing of the heart, represented on the ECG tracing by a pacemaker spike followed by a P wave or QRS complex

cardiac output: amount of blood ejected from the left ventricle per minute; normal value is 4 to 8 L/minute

cardioversion: restoration of normal rhythm by electric shock or drug therapy

carotid sinus massage: manual pressure applied to the carotid sinus to slow the heart rate

circus reentry: delayed impulse in a one-way conduction path in which the impulse remains active and reenters the surrounding tissues to produce another impulse

compensatory pause: period following a premature ventricular contraction during which the heart regulates itself, allowing the sinoatrial node to resume normal conduction

conduction: transmission of electrical impulses through the myocardium

conductivity: ability of one cardiac cell to transmit an electrical impulse to another cell

contractility: ability of a cardiac cell to contract after receiving an impulse

couplet: pair of premature beats occurring together

defibrillation: termination of fibrillation by electrical shock

deflection: direction of a waveform, based on the direction of a current

depolarization: response of a myocardial cell to an electrical impulse that causes movement of ions across the cell membrane, which triggers myocardial contraction

diastole: phase of the cardiac cycle when both atria (atrial diastole) or both ventricles (ventricular diastole) are at rest and filling with blood

ECG complex: waveform representing electrical events of one cardiac cycle; consists of five main waveforms (labeled P, Q, R, S, and T), a sixth waveform (labeled U) that occurs under certain conditions, the PR and QT intervals, and the ST segment

ectopic beat: contraction that occurs as a result of an impulse generated from a site other than the sinoatrial node

electrical axis: direction of the depolarization waveform as seen in the frontal leads

enhanced automaticity: condition in which pacemaker cells increase the firing rate above their inherent rate

excitability: ability of a cardiac cell to respond to an electrical stimulus

extrinsic: not inherently part of the cardiac electrical system

indicative leads: leads that have a direct view of an infarcted area of the heart

intrinsic: naturally occurring electrical stimulus from within the heart's conduction system

inverted: negative or downward deflection on an ECG

late electrical potentials: cardiac electrical activity that occurs after depolarization; predisposes the patient to ventricular tachycardia

lead: perspective of the electrical activity in a particular area of the heart through the placement of electrodes on the chest wall

monomorphic: form of ventricular tachycardia in which the QRS complexes have a uniform appearance from beat to beat

multiform or multifocal: type of premature ventricular contractions that have differing QRS configurations as a result of their originating from different irritable sites in the ventricle

nonsustained ventricular tachycardia: ventricular tachycardia that lasts less than 30 seconds

pacemaker: group of cells that generates impulses to the heart muscle or a battery-powered device that delivers an electrical stimulus to the heart to cause myocardial depolarization

paroxysmal: episode of an arrhythmia that starts and stops suddenly

polymorphic: type of ventricular tachycardia in which the QRS complexes change from beat to beat

preload: stretching force exerted on the ventricular muscle by the blood it contains at the end of diastole

proarrhythmia: rhythm disturbance caused or made worse by drugs or other therapy

quadrigeminy: premature beat occurring every fourth beat that alternates with three normal QRS complexes

reciprocal leads: leads that take a view of an infarcted area of the heart opposite that taken by indicative leads

reentry mechanism: failure of a cardiac impulse to follow the normal conduction pathway; instead, it follows a circular path

refractory: arrhythmia that doesn't respond to usual treatment measures

refractory period: brief period during which excitability in a myocardial cell is depressed

repolarization: recovery of the myocardial cells after depolarization during which the cell membrane returns to its resting potential

retrograde depolarization: depolarization that occurs backward toward the atrium instead of downward toward the ventricles; results in an inverted P wave

rhythm strip: length of ECG paper that shows multiple ECG complexes representing a picture of the heart's electrical activity in a specific lead

Stokes-Adams attack: sudden episode of light-headedness or loss of consciousness caused by an abrupt slowing or stopping of the heartbeat

sustained ventricular tachycardia: type of ventricular tachycardia that lasts longer than 30 seconds

systole: phase of the cardiac cycle when both of the atria (atrial systole) or the ventricles (ventricular systole) are contracting

trigeminy: premature beat occurring every third beat that alternates with two normal QRS complexes

triplet: three premature beats occurring together

uniform or unifocal: type of premature ventricular contraction that has the same or similar QRS configuration and that originates from the same irritable site in the ventricle

vagal stimulation: pharmacologic or manual stimulation of the vagus nerve to slow the heart rate

Valsalva's maneuver: technique of forceful expiration against a closed glottis; used to slow the heart rate

Index

i refers to an illustration; t refers to a table.

i refers to an illustration; t refers to a table.

i refers to an illustration; t refers to a table.

Notes

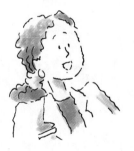

Notes

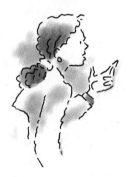

Notes

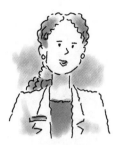

Notes

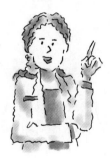

Notes

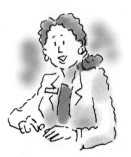

Notes

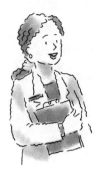